Half Man, Half M

As well as being a keen runner Mark I
multi-award-winning Future Toolbox, _ _____, _____
personal development for teenagers, young adults, schools, families
and community groups.

He and his wife Jules have written other titles including Don't Get
Your Neck Tattooed - The Z to A of Life Skills You Don't Get From
Sitting Exams, What the Hell Just Happened? and We All Follow The
Cobblers Over Land and Sea.

You can follow Mark and Jules on Facebook, Instagram, TikTok and
Twitter @kennedyauthors.

———

Half-man, Half-Marathon' is a fascinating look into the life of a runner
- why they do the seemingly crazy challenges and distances they do,
and what makes running so special. If you love running, you're going
to love this book.'

**Craig Lewis, Producer and presenter of the Running Tales
Podcast**

'Mark's book is both inspirational and funny and shows us all how
willpower, hope and the sense of being part of something special can
overcome all'

**Simon Hollis, Race Director Go Beyond Challenge and Ultra
Marathon Runner**

Half Man, Half Marathon covers topics that will resonate with both
new and experienced runners alike and also draws in real-life stories
from other runners out in the field, as well as sharing plenty of useful
hints and tips in every chapter.

Rik Vercoe: Founder of the 100 Half Marathon Club

Also by Mark Kennedy

Don't Get Your Neck Tattooed:
The Z to A of Life Skills You Don't Get From Sitting Exams

What The Hell Just Happened:
From Brain Injury to Bereavement and Breast Cancer

We All Follow The Cobblers… Over Land & Sea:
Stories Told By The Fans

Smarten Your Study:
How to Make Revision and Study, Easy and Fun

Available on Amazon, Kindle Unlimited and via our website
www.kennedyauthors.co.uk

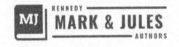

KENNEDY
MJ MARK & JULES
AUTHORS

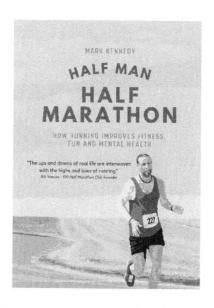

Half Man, Half Marathon

How running improves fitness, fun and mental health

Mark Kennedy

First published in 2022 in the UK

Future Toolbox
NN1 3PX

A catalogue number for this book is available from the British Library

ISBN 978-1-7391188-0-8

Cover design and illustrations: Admin and More

www.adminandmore.co.uk

For Thea, Isaac, Hugo and Oscar

Keep running towards
your goals

Mark
:)

Contents:

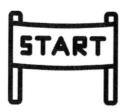

I. The Start Line

Running saved my life! Yes, this is a bold statement but it's true. It's a passion and a sport that has challenged me. It's pushed me past my comfort zone and beyond my limits. It's beaten me up and spat me out, but it also saved my sanity and my soul. It's given me goals and a focus, plus kept me fit. It's built my resilience and helped my mental health when I've been at a low point in my life. Most of all, it's forged some lifelong, solid friendships and bonds within a community of like-minded people. Simply put, I love running!

Like many people, running was something you did at the school cross country or in PE lessons and then you probably stopped once you left school. Your PE teacher shouted at you as you huffed and puffed around the field in the freezing cold.

I was always fit and active and walked absolutely everywhere. I would spend weekends with both of my grandparents, and we'd go on long walks. My nan would take me to the many parks and green spaces in Northampton, and we'd walk for miles. She always said that she stopped taking my pram from an early age because she'd end up pushing it with a shopping bag in the seat. My other nan and pap (pap is the Northampton dialect for grandpa) also loved our outdoor treks, and we'd drive out to the countryside and go on long walks. The family Sunday dinner was usually followed by a long walk before the adults would have 'five minutes'. This was a power nap on the sofa or chair. My mum also shared this love of going for a long walk too so, I guess being on my feet was ingrained into my DNA from an early age.

At school, I was the quiet, shy one who never really got into trouble. In my studies, I was generally in the middle of the group, never a highflyer but never in the bottom set. I guess I was often left to my own devices because I was the nice kid. Daydreaming was probably my specialised subject, and, if there were a grade for it, I'd have achieved top marks. That probably explains where my creativity came from. I loved art and creative writing. Anything that used my vivid imagination was a joy. As an only child, I was always happy to lose myself in my mind but, on the other hand, I was also sociable and loved talking to adults to find out how things worked. I'd also spend hours in my nan's garden, which seemed huge back then, and kick a football around pretending to be a top-flight player. That was amazing because I didn't have to worry about ability. I could win every game I imagined in my head and end up the top goal scorer.

As far as sport went, I never really excelled at that either and never got picked for any of the school sports teams. I was even called rubbish by some of my classmates and mocked a few times by a PE teacher. School can be a cruel place as kids are usually brutally honest with each other. Sometimes this didn't bother me as I kept myself to myself. Still, at other times it did knock my confidence. It meant I avoided anything that involved winning any competition or something that meant being in the limelight. I was happy sitting on the side-lines and being the quiet kid. I was always happy to be in the audience rather than on stage. There is a huge irony that I'm now a public speaker and love nothing more than standing on stage in front of hundreds of people. How that happened, I don't know! Also, as much as my family loved walking, none of them excelled at sports or were fiercely competitive. My mum was a swimmer and even had Olympic dreams as a teen but stopped competitive swimming before I was born.

My first experience of running in an event was at lower school. In the fourth year, our classes were entered into a sponsored run for charity. We had to pledge how many laps of the school field we'd run and then get our families to sponsor us an amount per lap. I pledged ten pence a lap and said I would do ten laps. My teacher uttered the words, 'Don't be silly, that's too far to run in that time!' My friend and I managed twelve laps!

It didn't really ignite my confidence in running though. I would stay in the confines of safely imagining I was winning a race. On family holidays to Bournemouth with my nan, aunty, uncle and cousins, I'd concoct a race from the promenade on Southbourne beach up the zig-zag path to the cliff top as we made our way home at the end of a busy day of building sandcastles, paddling in the sea and eating cheese sandwiches. I was the eldest of three cousins, so I'd invariably win the imaginary races. Over thirty years later, I still run with my cousin Sara at our running club and local parkruns, and we have fond memories of those childhood days.

In middle school, I volunteered to go to the cross-country club after school on a Monday night. I have absolutely no idea why as I didn't have any friends who joined. Perhaps it was following my glorious, sponsored run at Cedar Road Lower School a few months earlier. We ran a loop around the school fields on the first night there, and I came last. Undeterred, I went back and continued to finish last until Mr. O'Neill, the teacher, devised a handicap system to make it fairer. Each runner got a head start of the football pitch length based on their position. Of course, I got to go first, and that broke my streak of coming last. I don't remember why cross-country stopped; perhaps I gave up going, or maybe the evenings disbanded, but I don't remember running for a very long period. By the way, Mr. O'Neill was one of the most encouraging and excellent teachers. He was my form tutor in the third year at the school, and I have fond memories of attending his classes. It was a wonderful school, and I still see Mr. O'Neill, or Graham as I now address him, at football matches as we both support our local team.

As a football-mad kid, I was obsessed with stats, players, teams, fixtures, kits, names of football grounds and scores. I knew so much useless information about the sport it was unreal. I also watched my local team Northampton Town, home and away and am still a season ticket holder, where I see Graham, my former teacher of course.

So, how did running become a massive part of my life?
Well, it was by accident really. I was in my early thirties, and another one of my cousins, Ben, had entered the Great North Run and asked if I fancied a go. One of our friends had also entered but had to pull out due to injury and said I could run in her place. With only six weeks until the event, I politely declined as I wouldn't have enough time to train to run that far. However, the seed had been planted, and I committed to running the Great North Run the following year.

Fast forward to the present day, and running is more a part of my life than football. Yes, I still do a spreadsheet of my races and log my times and finish places. I count my training miles but not as full-on as I did with those football stats. One thing this gave me was a goal. That goal was to reach the 100 Half Marathon Club something I did in November 2021, and I was able to share the milestone with some fantastic friends. It certainly wasn't a lifelong ambition, it just happened to fall into my mind when I'd been running for a few years.

Running is incredible.
You hear tales of people running the length of the country or across desserts for days. Some runners do hundreds of back-to-back marathons for days on end, or complete ultra-distances week in, week out. We have Olympians who smash world records and run paces that most of us can just about achieve when driving our cars. Then there are the parkrunners, the couch to 5K groups, the first timers, the old-timers, the weight loss crew and the weekend warriors. Running is something that has grown in popularity in recent years and is more and more accessible to the population of the world. It's a community and a way of life.

The title of this book is Half Man, Half Marathon, based on my love of the 13.1-mile distance. I'd like to share with you some stories of running and positive mental health benefits that occurred to me on my journey one that was formed by simply putting one foot in front of another. It's something that has literally changed my life for the better, and I've witnessed it do the same for many others too.

So, lace up your trainers and get ready to enjoy my journey, and thank you for reading my stories. I hope some resonate with fellow runners or encourage a new runner to give this fantastic sport a chance. On your marks, get set... go!

2. The Best Day Gone Wrong

I wake up on the sofa in the conservatory, still wearing my running kit. There's the sound of plates rattling in the kitchen as my wife, Jules, is putting the washing up away in the cupboards. A slight breeze comes in through the open conservatory door as the hot autumn sun shines through the cracks in the blinds. I close my eyes again, trying to go back to sleep but I can't. Sitting upright, I stare at my running shorts and decide it's time to change. Now standing, I feel dizzy, and the world is spinning. I pass Jules on my way through the kitchen and head upstairs to change. She asked me how I feel, and I mutter a few words, '*still rough!*'

An hour or so later, I woke up lying on the bed. I looked down and I've still got the same running shorts on. The clock says it's approaching 5pm, and I feel more tired than when I woke in the conservatory. Sitting up, the room starts to spin, and I become breathless as if I've just sprinted for the finish line in a race. It worsened as I began hyperventilating, and a huge anxious feeling caused my arms and legs to shake uncontrollably. It felt awful!

Why would I have a panic attack right now? Nothing stressful or remotely dangerous is happening on this early September Sunday. My arms and legs felt like jelly, and I struggled to breathe. The whole world was blurred, and I couldn't focus on anything.

The Day Started So Well

That morning, I was buzzing to be lining up to run the Northampton Half Marathon, which started right in the town centre. It also coincided with the ska band Madness playing at The County Ground, home of Northamptonshire County Cricket Club. Best of all, both were within walking distance of my house. Buzzing was an understatement!

Have you ever had one of those days where everything should be so great, but it ends up being one of the worst days ever? This was one of them.

The race was wonderful until mile 10. For no apparent reason, I was physically sick. I started to walk, but something didn't feel right. It was like a fog in front of my face, and I couldn't breathe properly. I ran again, but the breathing became harder, so I stopped and sat on a grass verge at mile 11. A very kind volunteer walked down from the drink station, offered me a cup of water, and checked if I was OK. I smiled bravely and got to my feet after drinking the water. *'Only a couple of miles to go'*, I said. I started running, but the fog in front of me got foggier, and my legs wouldn't go where I wanted them to. The only option was to start walking again.

A car pulled up beside me, and a really friendly chap leaned across his seat and offered me a lift. Again, I smiled and politely declined and carried on walking. Two more kind-hearted strangers offered me lifts, but I somehow dug in and finished. I was determined not to drop out but had to walk past friends supporting me near the finish line. There were many concerned faces, but I just wanted to get to the end. One of the worst parts was the last few hundred metres when I saw some fellow runners from another club. They were out to support everyone on the day. As I passed them, they commented in jest, telling me to hurry up and get to the finish line. It was said in good spirits, but I felt I'd failed by walking at that stage. The thought that I'd dug in and finished instead of pulling out didn't seem like a victory.

I managed to run the final few steps over the line, was presented with my finishers medal, and then made a beeline for the biggest tree and hid in the woods, away from all my running friends. I felt so low, so I skipped the pub and somehow walked home.

It was then that I fell asleep in the conservatory and later found myself having one of the biggest panic attacks in my life in the bedroom that afternoon. The room was spinning, and my breath was attached to the back of my throat. I felt as if I was screaming but was lying on the bed hyperventilating. The strangest thing about it all was, I had no idea why! Absolutely no idea what had caused this! The day was exciting and not stressful, so why the avoidance?

I managed to get changed and forced myself out of the door to go to watch Madness but the world around me was still spinning. Naturally, Jules had been excited about meeting with friends pre-gig as the area was buzzing. However, I was now beating myself up for ruining everyone's day and my own, including my dream of running in the first Northampton Half Marathon. We stood at the back of the arena as Madness finished their final song of the set and I was shaking and close to tears. Why? Because I was struggling mentally to hold it together. My head was still foggy, and I could barely stand up. This was nothing to do with over-indulging in the spirit of the day by drinking too much, I just broke physically and emotionally that day.

How did this happen? You may be forgiven if you think that running 13.1 miles had perhaps sapped away my energy and caused me to flag out at home, but nothing could be further from the truth. This was, in fact, my 36th half marathon, and I'd been running for more than six years. I was fit, active and trained regularly, and the half was my favourite distance.

You may be familiar with my story, which Jules and I shared in our last book, *What The Hell Just Happened?* Just over a year before, in August 2012, I suffered a head injury in a freak accident while on holiday. I'd blacked out in a toilet in a small tapas bar and hit the right side of my head. Upon returning to England, I went to the hospital and was told that more than 90% of people don't survive that level of injury. I had a massive haematoma and a fractured skull on the right side of my head. There was also a smaller blood clot on the left side where my brain had hit the opposite side of my skull in the impact and had been dislodged. Yes, all this from a trip to the toilet!

However, as fate would have it, eight weeks after the impact I was signed off by the hospital, told it was a miracle and encouraged to live my life as normal. So, I did just that.

My first questions were about what I could do and what shouldn't I do. Sports-wise, I was told no to football and yes to running but, only a light jog. I quickly resigned myself to the fact I wouldn't be able to run a half marathon called the Beast in Dorset a week later. I opted for a gentle parkrun instead and felt great.

The thing is, I didn't realise the long-term effects of a brain injury include chronic fatigue, short-term memory issues and the inability to focus and concentrate for long periods. This cocktail of lasting effects causes low mood, high anxiety, mood swings and, worst of all, depression. I still struggle to use these terms as pre-brain injury I was pretty laid back, unfazed by anything and completely spontaneous most of the time.

Research and specialists had led me to believe that life would begin to return to normal after six months to a year. This episode at the Northampton Half was over a year later, and mentally, I felt ten times worse.

Looking back on this moment, I was delighted to be signed off, but I was offered no support. Physically, I had no signs of the accident, so the phrase *'hidden disability'* wasn't even a consideration.

Running and music were two things I loved and meeting up with friends at a local event was the ideal combination for a fantastic experience. How could I be in such a state? I didn't want to feel like this, but I found myself avoiding people and situations where I'd typically thrive. Yes, I have had poor runs in the past and been able to put them behind me and move on, but this was a big difference.

The day after the half marathon, Jules suggested I go to the doctor and seek advice. After a short period of procrastination, I did and was referred to the neurology department at Northampton General Hospital. The neurologist said to Jules, *'You just want your husband back, don't you?'* She nearly cried, and I felt like falling through the floor. The feeling of letting family and friends down and being a real drain on everyone was etched firmly in my mind, and I had no idea how to climb out of this deep hole of despair. Even today, I still struggle to write this paragraph with the memory of how broken I felt. Jules and I had been married for ten years and had an amazing relationship. Life was fabulous and could be described as almost perfect. Brain injury had changed my personality, and I was becoming a person I didn't want to be. I didn't like being withdrawn and stressed easily at times. Anxiety and grief would wash over me like a wave.

Life should've been good. I was fit and active and had survived a life-threatening injury. I was doing a job I loved as a self-employed freelance motivational speaker, travelling to schools all over the country. I was running for fun, we loved to travel, see live bands and lived in a beautiful house. Our friends were amazing, and life was good. The trouble is, I couldn't work out why it wasn't.

I did what most people would do in this situation, put on a brave face and tried my best to suppress the memories of that September day. A week later, I rocked up at my local parkrun and tried to run as hard as possible. The following week I came first in a Halloween Fun Run and decided to enter the Blenheim Half Marathon to exorcise the demons of Northampton.

Jules thought it was a good idea, and we drove to the beautiful palace in Oxfordshire. I had an excellent run, crossing the line in just over one hour and thirty-five minutes. We both hugged each other at the finish line, and I thought that I'd be able to move forward.

If only it were that easy though. I was getting good at the brave front but unable to follow up in the background. My running times were brilliant, but my recovery involved sleeping lots and feeling like I wanted to scream but couldn't. Can you relate to a time when your mouth is smiling, but your heart is aching? We're conditioned to keep calm and carry on, but it's not always that simple. Running seemed to be a big release, giving me time to lose the low thoughts. It forced me to be around people when running events, but I wouldn't have to have long conversations. A good run would usually be greeted with positive comments at the finish line, and I felt needy. This was great because running friends could compliment my running without me having to ask them to say something positive to me directly. This was working momentarily but wiping me out in the background.

Another trip to the doctors was met with the suggestion of trying a course of anti-depressants. I quickly dismissed that idea; after all, I wasn't depressed, which involved sitting at home and moping around. Having poor mental health means that I would be avoiding people and feeling the need to cry lots. Anxiety is one of those things that causes panic attacks, and none of those things applied to me. That's right, I was in denial too.

You probably don't need me to tell you that mental health is a hot topic in the world today. It's estimated that one in four adults will experience issues relating to mental health in their lifetime. However, I'm not here to give you loads of statistics and research, I just firmly believe that running and setting goals are one of many things that can promote positive mental health and well-being, and if it helps you too, then it's a win-win.

———

Stories From the Field - Real Life Runners

Throughout this book, I'll be sharing stories and lessons from fellow runners as well as my own. These will be real-life snippets into the lives of those who have found running to have a significant and positive impact on their lives.

———

Thoughts Running Through the Mind

This book is about more than just running, it's about life skills too. In 2009, Jules and I created a personal development company, Future Toolbox, and I will share some tools and tips with you at the end of each chapter. We all carry around a virtual toolbox and collect tools, which are knowledge, experience and wisdom. The more tools we have, the more we can expand and grow in our lives.

Since sustaining my brain injury, personal development has become even more important to me than ever before. Creating positive daily habits and working towards goals, has massively helped my recovery journey and helped me achieve the big life goals too. So, enjoy the tips in the, Thoughts Running Through the Mind sections and add them to your Future Toolbox.

Here goes with the first thoughts. In my first Northampton Half Marathon, things went far from the desired plan. So, think about when you expected something to be great, and it wasn't. It doesn't have to be as traumatic as my example above, which led to a full-on panic attack. How did you bounce back and learn to become more resilient?

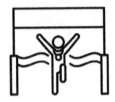

3. Crossing the Line

The crowd were cheering as I turned the corner, dropped down a slight slope and headed past the 12-mile marker. The sun was shining off the sea on the right-hand side and the noise was immense. It's almost as if someone had turned the volume up a notch. Looking up, I could see the finish line in sight. My legs were carrying me on adrenaline as I passed the 800 metres to go sign, then 400... and then the finish arch came into view.

A sharp turn onto a small grassy stretch, I threw my arms into the air as I crossed the line. It was a moment to cherish forever, and I felt like a superstar. Honestly, some 11,500 people had already crossed the line before me and twice that would follow, but I didn't care. It was my moment.

I mentioned, in the introduction, the conversation with my cousin Ben; well, a year later, I'd done it! It was the end of September 2007, and I'd done it. I'd completed my first ever half marathon, The Great North Run.

The Beginnings

Let me take you back in time to where it all began. These were pre-brain injury days when life was fun and spontaneous, and I was always up for a challenge. Until the previous year, my idea of fun was playing football and going to the gym. Running had always been one of those things that I thought would be boring or, dare I say it? Cliquey!

As mentioned, my cousin Ben and a couple of friends had done the Great North the previous year and suggested I give it a go. It sounded like a great idea, and I knew the event was something special.

I met a girl from the Northeast in the early nineties and ended up living in Newcastle for a few years. The locals used to go mad for the Great North Run, but I'd only ever seen it on TV. For some reason, her family said they'd been there, had seen it, and had no desire to go and watch it again. It was a shame because I'd have loved to have seen what all the fuss was about. Anyhow, now was my chance as I'd now entered the race.

Unfortunately, after Ben completed his race, he decided not to enter again after having a problem with his knee, so I did what most people do. Procrastinated! Should I do it or not? Hmm, I couldn't decide. It's a long way to run, and I'd have to train. Also, it might get in the way of playing football, and would I have to stop going to the pub? What about eating properly? Oh, and it's a long way to run…hold on, I've said that one already. As you can see, all the excuses were coming thick and fast, so I put it out of my mind.

February arrived, and I was sitting at work one day surfing the internet during a break. For some reason, I decided to check out the Great North Run website. It led me to some charity places, and one was for Cancer Research UK. I clicked through the link and learned I had to raise £400 for the charity. It sounded doable, but then the nagging doubt came back, could I run 13.1 miles? As far as I was concerned, running seemed a serious sport and only highly trained athletes who ran and ran and ran could do something like that. However, it was time for the acid test. I had a meeting with a mortgage adviser that evening after work. It was roughly a mile away. If I could run there without stopping, I'd enter the Great North Run.

The clock ticked past 5:30pm. I'd packed up my work stuff and headed out the door. Gingerly looking around, I made sure nobody was watching and I broke into a light jog along the main street through the town centre.

Have you ever felt unsuitably dressed for the moment? Well, that was me. Here I was in my work shoes, shirt and trousers with a coat on, running through town. I generally didn't care what other people thought, but I felt slightly stupid. The street was pedestrianised, so I couldn't even pretend I was running for a bus. Anyway, I had my goal in mind and reached my final destination, the mortgage adviser's office. Even with the road crossing, I hadn't stopped once and felt fine. It was time to compose myself, wipe the sweat away and climb the stairs. I later learned that Studney, that mortgage adviser, was also a runner and we've become good friends since.

The following day, I realised that there was no turning back. I called Great Run, pledged to raise £400 for Cancer Research UK and paid my entry fee. That was it, no more excuses, I was doing the Great North Run.

I was excited and wanted to get started on my training plan. There was an inner belief that I could actually do it. With around seven months to train, the first step was to go for a proper run. I popped on an old pair of trainers, some football shorts and a gym top and headed to the park. Abington Park was the scene of one of the Northampton School for Boys cross country runs in PE lessons. Our PE teachers would take us on a lap of the school field and then we'd head out into the streets and do a lap of the park. It was a killer for a teenager, but it was time to see how I'd fare as a thirty-something bloke.

My goal was to run a lap without stopping. After getting out of the car, selecting a track on my MP3 player and looking around gingerly, I set off. The first stretch was downhill, and as the cold air hit my lungs, I soon got into a stride, and it felt great. Not only did I manage a lap, I did two. So delighted, I got in the car and drove around the park to measure the distance. It was 3.2 miles! That was it; my training had officially started.

A few days after signing up for the Great North Run, a glossy brochure arrived in the post. It was from Cancer Research and included a training plan on the back page. It had beginners, intermediate and advanced versions. I was fortunate to be starting with a three-mile run under my belt, so I opted for the intermediate. Then I saw the long runs, and some were in double figures. This was quite daunting, even though I knew I had to run 13.1 miles. It was time to get a bit serious as this wouldn't be an easy challenge.

Cotton Vest, Black Trainers and Safety Pins! It's Getting Serious!

The old trainers I'd run in were barely good enough to walk in, and my feet started to hurt after a few more laps of the park, so it was time to invest in a new pair. I headed to a sports shop chain in town and bought a black pair of trainers for £20. They looked like they'd do the job and proved more comfortable as I began to up my training distance.

Sid, a mate from my football team, suggested a local 10K event and I decided to enter. It was at Silverstone Circuit, which is a short drive from home. The idea of running around the home of the British Grand Prix was quite appealing. Like the Great North Run, racing at Silverstone was something I'd only seen on television.

I was armed with my black trainers, football shorts and a cotton vest. I mean, you must wear a vest for running, don't you?

As my wife, Jules, and I hopped in the car, Jules did her usual, have you got everything check. The one thing we realised that was missing from the list was safety pins. Oh yeah, I'd be wearing a number and how else would I attach it to my vest?

We drove to the little corner shop, and I asked the guy behind the counter if he sold safety pins. Half expecting to get an answer of, why on earth do you think I'd sell safety pins, he surprised me by producing a little plastic bag full of them and asked how many I wanted. Bizarre, but there wasn't much that this guy didn't sell. I think I bought the minimum amount, probably about ten of them, pinned to a little piece of card. Arriving at Silverstone, I soon learned that you don't need to buy your own pins as there were boxes with thousands of them in there. I now probably own enough to set up my own safety pin shop if there's such a market.

It was race time and I was ready. Well, as ready as I'd ever been. Looking around, there were so many serious-looking people sprinting up and down the pit lane. They were wearing running club vests and proper running shoes. Have you ever had one of those moments where you feel seriously out of your depth? Well, this was it for me. Nobody was wearing black trainers and I couldn't see many cotton vests. Trying to fit in, I casually did the good old quad stretch. Leaning against the wall, I pulled my right heel towards my backside and puffed my chest out attempting to look confident. Inside I felt a little nervous, but I was sure I wasn't the only first-timer here. In all honesty, most of the serious runners were probably engrossed in their own race preparations, and the newer runners focused on their own nerves.

As Jules was pinning my number on my vest and I was moving onto the left leg stretch, Sid made his way through the crowd, looking suitably dressed for the occasion. He had a pair of white running shoes on and a running t-shirt. Suddenly I felt a bit more relaxed. It was the sight of a friendly face.

Jules gave me a good luck hug and hugged Sid before telling him to look after me. We then made our way to that start line among the thousand or so other runners.

I had no plan, so I stuck with Sid, and we chatted as the race began. The pace was surprisingly comfortable as we passed the 1km marker. The pre-race nerves and imposter syndrome feeling started to disappear.

At the end of the first lap, Jules was cheering us both on; that was a special moment. I waved like a lunatic as we passed the 5km point and approached the water station. A guy handed me a cup of water which I attempted to drink but spilt most of it down my cotton vest. It was a moment where I tried to style it out, conscious that the cheering crowd would begin laughing. For you runners out there, you'll have experienced this often.

We got to 9km, and Sid asked me how I was feeling. At this point, I'd gone a little quieter and was struggling a little with the pace. He decided to push on to the finish line and I encouraged him to continue. As he disappeared into the crowd of runners, I dug in and decided to get to the end without stopping. The final kilometre seemed longer than the previous nine, but I managed to sprint the last hundred metres and crossed the line feeling good. My little stopwatch said 47:45. At that point, I'd stopped caring about all those serious runners in their running colours and those white running shoes. Also, nobody had the faintest idea that I'd bought my own safety pins from the newsagents either. In fact, everyone was running their own race in their own zone. I later discovered that I'd finished about halfway in a field of just under a thousand runners. My running event journey had now begun.

I'm Never Going to Walk Again
The training plan for the Great North Run was displayed on the kitchen cupboard and each run was ticked off with the time it took to complete. This was quite a feat as I'm usually a kind of wing it guy. You know, make it up as you go along? Following a training plan gave me the discipline to work towards my goal of that daunting 13.1 miles.

Each training run would consist of spending a few minutes on a website called MapMyRun to plot the route. This was an excellent tool for my planning because I could now work out where I was going and how far specific points and landmarks were. Nowadays, many apps and GPS running watches map your route and tell you your pace, distance and all sorts of other stats. I didn't own any of this gear, so it involved a little extra work. I'd lace up the black trainers and head out the door in my cotton vest and football shorts.

At times I'd get someone quoting Forest Gump and shouting '*Run Forest run*' as I headed along the streets, but I began to stop caring about this sort of stuff. Running seemed quite natural and felt quite effortless at times. Friends would comment and say I was built for running. I'm never sure how the science of genetics works, but being tall and slim, I guess I fit the bill.

Occasionally, a truck driver would bellow out, '*run fat boy, run*,' in reference to the Simon Pegg film of the same name, that had been recently released in 2007. Being '*built for running*,' I've never been overweight, so this just made me smile.

One lovely June evening, I was out for a post-work training run and headed to an area called the Washlands. One great thing about living in the centre of Northampton is that you're only a couple of miles from the countryside as the town is surrounded by green. I made my way along the riverbank, crossed a bridge and returned along the other side. As I reached a gravel path, I took my next step and suddenly, ouch! A pain shot through my knee. After a couple more steps, I stopped and stretched for a moment. Restarting my watch, I began jogging gingerly, but each time I put weight on the foot, the pain shot up my leg into my knee. I was gutted! Having no option, I turned around and started to walk home. Walking was fine, but every attempt to jog it out was met with the same pain.

As I wandered in the house, Jules asked me how my run had gone and, like a sad figure, I told her of the pain. I was comforted by her usual hug, but I sat, wondering if I'd ever walk again. In hindsight, I'd just walked a couple of miles now, so I guess it wasn't going to be that serious. However, I booked a doctor's appointment the following day to get my knee looked at.

Now, most people say to never go to the doctor with things like this because the doc will probably tell you to stop running. Our doctor was different though. He examined my knee and explained it was probably something called 'runners' knee', which is quite common in runners. I guess everything there makes sense! I'm running, and I have a knee, so, runner's knee. Yeah, simple really. He then asked me if I had the right running shoes. I explained the black trainers, and he suggested I invest in a proper pair. The next piece of advice was to rest for a week, and things should be fine.

So, I did what many male patients do after a visit to the doctor, listen and then ignore his advice. Firstly, I didn't need to pay silly amounts of money for these fancy shoes. Secondly, in football, we have a phrase that says 'run it off'. Fortunately, I have a very sensible and caring wife who suggested I rest for a week and perhaps invest in some proper running shoes. So, I decided to listen to one of those things and rested for a week. Thankfully, the knee pain subsided, and I resumed my training plan.

Breaking the Bank

What is it with these bloody shoes? At the time, a friend at work was a keen and serious runner, and she'd completed the London Marathon several times. She kept telling me to buy some decent running shoes. I'd done a couple of events, and everyone was wearing these expensive-looking trainers. I'd speak to people at the end of races and overhear conversations about running shoe brands. I'd also subscribed to Runners World, and every magazine was loaded with adverts for shoes.

Perhaps it was a combination of not being caught up in the hype of anything fashion or label related and being a bit of a tight arse when it comes to spending, but I still thought I could do without my running shoes. These black trainers will be fine I kept telling myself.

Have you ever had one of those days when something kicks you up the backside, and you feel that you should've listened? Well, that day arrived on another training run. I was just over a mile into the route before I took a tumble. Yep, running along a busy street with traffic lined up on either side of the main road and people going in and out of shops, the stage was set to look extremely stupid. I was bounding along, listening to some rock music on my headphones and enjoying the sunshine, when suddenly, I was flying through the air before the inevitable thud. Being a bloke full of bravado, I immediately jumped to my feet and glared at the very slightly raised paving slab. You know, the one where you're holding back from punching it or telling it what you really think of this inanimate object? A guy at the cash point shouted, 'You OK mate?' to which I replied I was and broke into a jog as if it was all part of the act.

After a couple of hundred metres, I realised blood was pouring down my leg and I decided to assess the damage. There was a small cut on my knee and both my elbows were grazed and bleeding. I also noticed a huge scuff on the front of my black trainers and a little hole just above my toes.

Looking like a wounded war hero, I decided to soldier on and complete my training run. On the way home, I passed the battle site where I'd sustained my bloody knees and elbows and decided to stop and survey the area. The offending paving slab was only raised a couple of millimetres, yet it had ruined my twenty-quid pair of shoes. *'Bloody slab, I'll give you what for'*, I muttered as I ran home and explained to Jules why my arms and knee were covered in blood.

It was time to give in, accept the world's advice and get myself a pair of running shoes. I headed to The Running Shop in Northampton. Yes, the shop was actually called that! And it did exactly what it said on the tin.

I wandered into the shop and browsed the shoes on the rack. Noticing a price tag of £130 for a pair, I immediately put that shoe down and scanned the prices. Everything seemed to be in three figures, a hundred and something pounds and I was breaking into a cold sweat. Perhaps I could return to the high street sports shop and buy another cheap pair.

Then a friendly lady appeared from the back of the shop and apologised that she hadn't heard the door open. I stated the obvious - that I needed a pair of running shoes. Showing her the pair I'd been running in, she gave the diagnosis that I certainly did need a better pair and asked if I'd mind running along the path outside so she could check my gait. I thought a gait was something that you opened and closed until I'd read something in Runners World. Again, not really buying into the hype of science, I'd sort of glossed over all this technical stuff. I mean running, you put one foot in front of the other and move faster than the walking pace. It can't be more complicated than that, surely?

After returning to the shop, the lady told me I was an over-pronator. I joked that it usually takes me a while to make decisions, but then I realised that was a procrastinator.

After chuckling, she explained, *'Pronating is to do with how your feet land, and you have a strong heel strike!'* I mentioned that I don't always buy into hype but love listening to experts and learning. After a conversation, I trusted this lady's judgement and knowledge and was ready to buy a pair of running shoes. She immediately walked over to the shelf and took down the £130 pair. Bloody hell, not those I thought, but I accepted that I needed to spend some money here. After trying on a couple of pairs, I was delighted that the pair that suited me best was £90 a pair. So, I became the owner of some Brooks running shoes. And they were white.

The Big Day, I Was Hooked

Finally, the weekend of the Great North Run arrived. Jules and I drove to Newcastle on the Saturday afternoon the day before the event. I felt calm and full of excitement about the race. We checked into our hotel in the coastal town of Whitley Bay, which was a short hop on the metro into Newcastle city centre. I knew Whitley Bay from my days up north and had found a place called Banana Grove. Yep, it was everything you expected from a place in a party street by the seaside. Two giant plastic palm trees were outside the bar that sat beneath the rooms. The receptionist offered us a drink discount voucher in the bar, and we went downstairs to catch some evening football on the TV. Jules was at the bar ordering me a shandy and enquiring about the game being on when I noticed a stripper emerge from backstage and begin her clothes-removing routine. This was one thing I didn't remember about my nights out in Whitley Bay. A few fellow runners also stood at the bar, their jaws dropping at the sight that greeted them. We politely decided to leave as this wasn't the ideal race preparation.

The whole day was magic from start to finish. I had absolutely no nerves at all. Runners in fancy dress, themed t-shirts, charity outfits, and of course, serious running attire too, lined the pavements. There were even people in cotton vests and black trainers. The place was buzzing. We stood on a raised bank in the sunshine and watched the ladies' race start, with Olympian and then Marathon World Record Holder Paula Radcliffe leading the field. I then got my usual good luck hug from Jules and made my way to my starting point in Pen D. Big events have sections for runners based on their predicted finish time to try and ease the congestion on the course. I was now squeezing between runners of all shapes and sizes, and suddenly, the sport had a whole different meaning. It wasn't cliquey, there was a sense of togetherness.

The race was started by former England manager Sir Bobby Robson, someone I was a massive fan of. I was excited to catch a glimpse of him on a giant big screen as the countdown began from ten. The crowd joined in... nine, eight, seven, six... and the excitement around me rose... five, four, three, two, one... gooooooo! And suddenly, we went nowhere! Yep, there were a few thousand people in front of me who needed to cross the start line before my race could start.

Suddenly, a ripple of laughter went around the crowd of runners. Looking up at the big screen, we could see some goon who'd managed to get into the elite section and sprinted off into a lead of about thirty metres. At least he could say he led the Great North Run for a while.

After a few minutes of shuffling forward, I crossed the start line and quickly settled into a comfortable pace. A mile or so in, the course crosses the Tyne Bridge, and the next thing I heard was the unbelievable roar of the

Red Arrows overhead. Turning into Gateshead, on the opposite side of the River Tyne, I overheard a guy warn his mate that we were approaching the hill. To be honest, I didn't notice the incline, I was too busy enjoying the passionate crowds and bands dotted around the course, playing songs from The Blaydon Races to Highway to Hell.

Suddenly I passed a sign saying halfway and pulled my mobile phone out of my pocket to text Jules to tell her where I was on the course. Mastering running while drinking a cup of water was one thing, but texting was another.

At 11 miles, I saw two guys giving out their home-brewed beer. Many people had said to look out for them, but I was in the middle of the road and far too nervous to consider beer and running simultaneously.

'Go on Cobblers Mark' came the cheers from the Cancer Research bus in the final mile. I felt like a celeb, wearing the charity t-shirt with my name on it. The Cobblers part comes from Northampton Town Football Club, the team I support. They're known as The Cobblers from the town's shoemaking history.

I collected my medal after crossing the line and felt like a winner. Time and time again, I'd visualised this moment in my head. Running 13.1 miles had previously seemed like an impossible, far-out dream, but it was now a reality. As the Red Arrows flew over the North Sea and the sunshine reflected off the ripples of the water, I stood there with Jules and just enjoyed the moment. It was time to celebrate.

We made our way back to the metro station in South Shields only to be greeted with the world's biggest queue. So, we headed to the pub for a celebratory pint and swapped stories with fellow runners.

I sat there and began sending text messages to family and friends who'd sponsored me and then started receiving replies asking what on earth I was talking about. Instead of forwarding the message that I'd done the Great North Run, I somehow managed to message everyone the word omeprazole, which was a medication my dad had suggested for digestion. After realising the error, I re-texted everyone to tell them I'd done it.

———

Stories From the Field - Real Life Runners: First Time

We usually have a strong memory of the first time we did something. I talked to some of my fellow local runners and asked them how they felt the first time they completed a race.

Laura did her first-ever 10K at a beautiful stately home. She said, '*I felt like I was superwoman, overcome with emotion and pride... then I was given a travel mug instead of what should have been my first ever medal and I cried. Oh, the* tears were sheer overwhelming disappointment at the fact I got a travel mug and not the medal I'd dreamed of my entire life!'

Jason's first run was a five-mile event quite a few years back. He said, 'After crossing the finish line, my thoughts were, I love all the people cheering me on. Did I win something?'

Lesley completed a 5KM event, stumbling over the finish line and crying, 'I felt so proud I had completed it, I will never forget that feeling.'

Theresa did her first-ever event, a 10K in Milton Keynes, in February 2020. 'I remember it was in the tail end of Storm Dennis. I was wet through and cold but so proud and happy and blissfully unaware it would be my last 'proper' event for a long time as we all know what happened not long after that!' Indeed, the pandemic was just around the corner and took away many things we loved doing.

Dan shared his story! 'My first road race was Northampton Half Marathon in 2019. I was running for charity in my first race as a member of my new running club. I was utterly broken by mile seven, but through encouragement from some fellow members, who helped me up a killer hill and ran with me for three miles, I got through to the end and even managed a little sprint race to the finish line. I felt so happy, it was the furthest I had ever run, and to have done it for a very special charity, wearing the colours of a very special club, and the support of some very special people, I felt very lucky. An hour later, my legs refused to carry me anywhere.' Who said running is an individual sport, hey?

Mark said, 'I felt like I was a superhero, absolutely flying along in the last mile of my first half marathon, only to be serenely overtaken by Buzz Lightyear, who was being chased by Scooby Doo.' OK, just to be clear, they were fellow runners dressed as Buzz and Scooby Doo, not the real cartoon characters.

Bob is a man after my own heart. He loves a challenge and, despite suffering from a heart condition, he regularly runs half marathons and marathons. He's well on his journey to the 100 Half Marathon and 100 Marathon Clubs. Bob shared his beginnings and love of running. 'My first event was a local parkrun in January 2016. When I finished, apart from the relief of having completed it, I felt I could do better. Something that still happens now, but occasionally, I've cried and laughed with pride.'

Andy is retired, and he is running stronger than ever. He said those immortal words never again and then went back for more. 'The first time across the finishing line was the London Marathon. I got my medal from Jonathan Edwards, he looked at me as I said I'm never going to run another step in my life! He replied, give it an hour or so, you will change your mind! I guess he was right.' Andy now regularly bags Good for Age places in marathons, and he won't mind me using the cliche that he does look very good for his age. He also recently ran for England in the veteran masters. That's some achievement!

One of my club mates, Pete, recently ran his first ultra. He recalled the friendliness of his first-ever running event experience, *'My first ever race was Desborough 10K. After running with friends Bob, Louise and Gemma for a while, I was encouraged to enter this event. Bob gave me encouragement on the day, and I must admit I loved it. To cross the line was a brilliant feeling, and the addiction progressed. Louise reminded me that I wasn't sure if I wanted to be a runner or a cyclist, but I guess that was the moment I chose running. Initially, Bob, Louise and Gemma were complete strangers but soon became newly found friends via Tuesday Treacles running group. The plan was to improve running for sprint Triathlon events, but we've all achieved some amazing things since and, most importantly, have forged some strong friendships.'*

Some people pick a simple 5K fun run as their first race but not Alison. *'My first event was the Great Wall of China Half Marathon. I had a colic baby and insomnia and began running when he was two months old for my mental well-being. I would hand him to my husband as he walked in the door from work and out I went. One night while awake, I found this race online and messaged a friend saying I wanted to go. She said sure, and the training for the next six months kept me sane. I flew from Toronto to Beijing when my son was ten months old. They announced my name and country as I crossed the finish line and I felt like I was an Olympian. I was so happy, with tears. I had never been considered an athlete. I still feel awkward when referred to as an athlete, perhaps with imposter syndrome, but I suppose I am.'*

I met Steve a few years ago and he told me he took up running to get fitter and more active. Recently, we chatted about his first ever half marathon, which like mine, was the Great North Run. *'One Friday while eating a fast-food meal and entered the Great North Run. As my first ever running experience, it was exciting but scary. I'd never run before, never done a parkrun, didn't even have any trainers and didn't even know how far a half marathon was but what an experience it became. I stopped smoking, ate healthier, lost weight and most importantly, achieving that goal gave me enormous relief at that finish line. I realised that I could do things if I set my mind to it. That race was the catalyst for finding out I'm good at something and believing in myself. I go back to the Great North Run every single year as a pilgrimage, still with the same love and the same excitement. When I see some green bus shelters at mile ten, I'm still looking for that one lad that gave me an orange to 'make me run faster'.*

I think running, in general, is a huge lesson for anyone. There are times when you must learn resilience to push through difficult moments. Likewise, there are times when a run can be the most blissful part of your day when you feel all the stress melt from you, and it gives clarity of mind to help you find the solution or have a break from everything. Plus, it's one of the few sports where we are equal to a degree, as no matter what your pace or distance, we all started with that first *run and even the elites have experienced the same tough moments. I think that's why the rapport among runners is unique. We all get it; we have all had those moments, and the camaraderie among what can be total strangers really makes you feel part of a larger community and social circle'*

Finally, Roger, a very good mate and the chairman of our running club, Northampton Road Runners, said, '*I love every finish line. It always gives me a thrill and never gets boring. Occasionally, when I've pushed hard, I've had that 'close to passing out' feeling or chasing the clock until I burst, but mostly, each time I do it, it reminds me how lucky I am to be fit and healthy and able to do something so amazing.'*

I love that mindset and agree wholeheartedly. It's always a special moment, whatever the event.

———

Thoughts Running Through the Mind

I'm humbled hearing the stories of new runners finding their feet (no joke intended there). Have you ever stumbled upon something accidentally and realised how much you love it? Sometimes, we prejudge something we've yet to try, and when we open our minds, we realise it wasn't actually that bad after all.

Challenge yourself to try something new. Ask yourself, what have I been putting off or saying that I don't like, but, with a bit of practice or interaction, it might be something that I could enjoy or benefit from?

Now make a note of it and think about how or when you could try it. Perhaps it's a new food or one you tried years ago, but now you love it because your taste has changed.

Is there a hobby or pastime you've had a nagging urge to begin but haven't because it sounds hard to do, or perhaps time gets in the way? Maybe you could set a plan of how you could take this up as a new challenge.

Maybe there's a country or place you've wanted to visit, or if you dare to dream, move to and live in. A non-running friend of mine always wanted a pink house by the sea and moved to that pink house a few years ago. She simply removed all the barriers from her life and looked for ways to make it happen. How could you visit that dream place or take that leap of faith? Go on, start planning it now!

4. Beginners Guide to Running

'*You're not a failure; you just haven't quite succeeded as often as those with more practice have.*' Wow, what a quote! I heard someone say it recently and guess we all have this feeling of others being better than us, and that's OK when we're starting out.

So perhaps there is no beginner's guide. We all start as novices and must find our feet (ooh, it's that running metaphor again). I guess I didn't know what my benchmark was for my first 10K or half marathon, but I felt pleased with my times and being able to run the whole way without stopping. I found that my time was pretty reasonable for a newbie back then.

Since beginning my journey in 2007, running has changed massively, and we now have more beginners' groups, casual jogging groups, fun runs and parkrun. As I said before, I remember thinking running was quite elitist, but that stereotype seems to have lessened year upon year, thankfully. Speed isn't important and taking walking breaks is totally acceptable. However, we wouldn't be human if we didn't feel like an imposter from time to time. There are many common fears for newer runners so, I asked some of my fellow running club members what their fears included:

- What if I finish last?
- Everyone's looking at me.
- I'm too slow and I'm holding everyone back.
- I'm not the right shape for running.
- If I walk, then I've failed.
- Being caught up by fellow runners in an event.
- If I wear this club running vest, people will think I'm too serious a runner and I'm not.
- Getting leg cramps, stomach cramps or other pains.
- What if I have to drop out of a race or quit a training run?
- Will my health issues or mental health hold me back?
- Not being as quick as I used to be.

What surprised me was the self-conscious answers came from as many men as they did women. This was also from a range of beginners and experienced runners. And in fact, many experienced runners still have some of these anxieties from time to time.

A friend rightly pointed out, "We need to remind ourselves that we're one of 7.9 billion people. Who actually cares what we do or what we look like?"

It's true! How often do we sit there and judge other people out running, cycling, fishing, stamp collecting, potholing, sailing, mountain climbing, train spotting or whatever their pastime may be? Yet, this wave of self-consciousness has such a hold over us all.

A friend of mine has run around 200 marathons and has walked in almost every single one of them. And people who know him in the running community all think his achievements are incredible. You'll hear more from him later.

Another running buddy said, "I had a customer tell me once I wasn't the right shape for a runner, but it hasn't stopped me trying." And why should it? Does that customer get any benefit from your running? Of course not! Do they feel a sense of achievement when you cross the finish line? Nope!

To ensure my running club wasn't skewed with answers, I asked more runners from our local parkrun and other running groups, and the answers were the same. You could also make a solid bet that this goes for any other pursuit in life. Imposter syndrome has a lot to answer for, that's for sure.

When I began running, people said I was naturally gifted, but I certainly didn't feel like that. I remember doing a few 5K and 10K events, including my first at Silverstone, and feeling hugely self-conscious. I didn't feel really quick, even though my times were reasonable. I compared myself to others and, at times, still do. To date, I've completed ten marathons and have never broken four hours. Some people reading this would love to break five hours, six hours or even just complete a run, never mind a marathon. However, lots of people comment that they're surprised I've never done a sub-four-hour 26.2 event. It was a bit of a monkey on my back a few years ago until I shoved that chimp away and told it to do one. I don't really care anymore. I'm just grateful to have done those marathons. OK, being honest, part of me would still love to have that achievement on my running CV but it's fine.

Marathons aside, imposter syndrome has raised its head many times. Friends in events have beaten me, I've beaten myself up for not running well enough, I've had to walk when I've felt I should be running, my speed has dropped, and I've felt too serious at times. On top of that, mental health issues have sometimes eaten away at my running, and I've not been open and honest enough to admit that.

The Final Finishers

When I joined my running club, Northampton Road Runners, one thing that immediately struck me was the celebration of my fellow members. At my first cross country event, it was emotionally touching to see our top runners cheering on those finishing at the back of the field. This is an excellent ethos of our club, standing in the pouring rain and waiting for everyone to finish when others are eating cake.

This is another wonderful culture that has been brought into the limelight at parkruns all over the country. The average finish time gets slower each year, and this is wonderful. At our local parkrun, we have a legend called Bob, who's in his late eighties. Fellow runners feel a sense of connection when they see him on the course. With all respect to the runners who finish at the front, we don't see them until the end.

On that note though, the top local runners are incredibly humble too. They offer nothing but encouragement and love to their fellow athletes. Everyone runs their own race.

Comrades Marathon

The Comrades Marathon sums up the spirit of running. It's the world's oldest ultramarathon run over a 55-mile route in the KwaZulu-Natal province of South Africa. Each year, the course direction changes between Durban and Pietermaritzburg, and around 25,000 competitors participate in this gruelling event. On Wikipedia, the event description says, '*The spirit of the Comrades Marathon is said to be embodied by attributes of camaraderie, selflessness, dedication, perseverance, and ubuntu (which means humanity).*'

The event has a cut-off time of twelve hours, and any runner finishing after this point is officially out of the race. I remember reading an article in the Runner's World magazine talking about how the locals and spectators give the biggest cheer for the first person who crosses the line after the cut-off time has passed. This runner is the first unofficial runner whose hardcore effort isn't recorded, and they don't get presented with a medal. It's as if their race didn't exist. This person's effort is more celebrated than the winner. It's a wonderful thought.

Stories From the Field - Runners Getting Started

I've been running for long enough now to know that we all feel incredibly conscious of our own performances, even if we're the most experienced runners in the world. It was time to go out into the running community and ask some friends what they think and feel.

Rebecca admitted, '*Being slow still worries me, but I no longer care if people are looking and, if they ever were, running makes me feel great.*'

Sometimes things are beyond our control, and Kathy summed that up really well, '*I would worry about being slow and holding everyone back! But explaining why I'm much slower due to medical reasons has been empowering for me. I now have the confidence to go out with a group of runners since my life-changing events, which has really boosted my self-esteem.*'

Natasha was also worried about speed. '*I was running to shift a lot of pregnancy and lifestyle weight and was incredibly self-conscious about it. Once I rediscovered my love of running, I chose to ignore those voices in my head! It's amazing the pressure we put on ourselves.*'

James showed that running can bring many of its highs and lows at times, '*I sometimes feel that I'm trying to get back to the better version of my running self and not quite getting there. It's like all my best achievements are in the rear-view mirror!*'

Jane told me that she started running four days after having a baby. '*My biggest fear was literally peeing my pants.*'

When you chat with him, he seems very confident on the outside. In fact, Simon's first run was a 100-mile ultra that he was roped into as part of a work team. You'd think he'd be made of steel after that, but it was, in fact, the opposite. '*People looking at me used to be a big one until I remembered I'm not important, so why would people waste their time on someone they don't know? It's amazing how you can create these hang-ups in your own head sometimes. I've tried thinking about how much attention I pay to others when I'm out and about, and I can safely say it's not much.*'

Rob and John also dispelled a common misconception that blokes are competitive and confident. Rob said, '*I would worry that people would make fun of my little legs and knee on shorts and still not being good enough to keep up or keep going. Now I don't care what others think. I just enjoy my running and the friendships it's given me.*'

John echoed Rob's words, '*I was terrified of wearing shorts because of my skinny, white legs but soon found out that nobody really cares and now not wearing shorts would be so weird.*'

Both are excellent runners and respected locally. They've achieved some brilliant things, running events right up to the ultra-distance, but most of all, they're an inspiration to others around them. John helped a partially sighted runner achieve a sub-four-hour virtual marathon during the lockdown, and they've since become great friends that make a pair of shorts seem pretty insignificant. There's more on that story later.

———

Thoughts Running Through the Mind

What have you feared having a go at but then realised that you're good at something? Perhaps you've been conscious of looking silly in front of others and then realised people are celebrating your achievements.

Did you know that over 90% of things we worry about are unnecessary thoughts? More often than not, the things we fear never actually happen.

What if this goes wrong?
What if I don't like it?
What if I fail?
What happens if I break it?
What if people laugh at me?

Change those thoughts and flip your questions around. Try asking yourself:

How will I feel when it goes well?
How will I celebrate when I get it right and succeed?
What if I do like it?
Is it really that breakable, and even if it is, how can I fix it and learn from an error?
Who cares what others think? I'm going to do it anyway!

Remember that we all must learn to walk before we can run. A child never gives up when they fall after taking their first steps. They never look at their parents and feel self-conscious because they've been laughed at or tumbled and didn't get it right the first time. Ask yourself, what are my first steps towards my goal, and how can I take them?

The final thought to be mindful of, is perhaps we as humans should be less judgmental of others around us. I'll hold my hands up to poking fun at friends and even complete strangers on occasions in the past. Even banter can be taken the wrong way at times. We're all guilty of doing this and sometimes don't realise the impact it could have on someone's self-confidence and mental health.

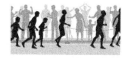

5. What Next? A Marathon?

The weeks after completing the Great North Run, I was buzzing. Everyone kept asking me the same questions.

'Are you doing the marathon next?!'
'What was your time?'
'Are you going to do it again next year?'
'Do you want your sponsorship money?'
'What's next?'

Friends wanted me to run London, but I kept playing it down. The thought of two half marathons on the same day seemed too far. Doing the Great North Run again did appeal to me. I'd also raised over £1,300 for Cancer Research in the process, more than three times my target, and my time was 1:59:37, which I was delighted with.

The nagging voice was there all the time. London, London, London. I went onto the London Marathon website and learned that race entry had closed. Sometimes that brings great relief because that means you don't have to do it. On the other hand, it further eggs on your desire to have something you can't have so I continued to look for ways of how to enter. Aha, a charity place could be the answer! I began scoring through the charity pages and sending emails to the biggies like the British Heart Foundation, Marie Curie, and of course, spoke to Cancer Research, whom I'd run the Great North for. I also tried some of the smaller, lesser-known organisations, but pretty much all had filled their places too.

While scrolling, I noticed a familiar logo, that of the YMCA. No, not anything to do with the Village People's hit; I mean the actual YMCA organisation. Now, let me explain why! At the time, Jules was the training manager for YMCA Training in Northampton, running a successful training centre that was linked to the local hostel.

I called the number in the advertisement and was half expecting the usual, '*Sorry, we've filled our quota*', response but the lady I spoke to gave me some great news. They had a couple of places left. She asked me for some information on my running and fundraising experience. The rapport was instant, and that was before I name-dropped Jules into the conversation. The application form was a simple formality, but I now had my place. Pledging to raise £1,300 in sponsorship seemed easier than running 26.2 miles. However, I was excited as I waited for the acceptance email. This arrived a day later, and the fundraising contact even agreed to allocate 40% of the funds raised to the Northampton YMCA. I was delighted, excited and nervous. Now I had to start training.

The day after being accepted, I received a call from the area director of the local YMCA welcoming me on board. He was honoured that I'd pledged some of my funds to the local part of the charity. It was a lovely personal touch which really meant a lot.

Another day passed, and my fundraising pack arrived with a booklet including tips on marathon training. I was excited until I read the training schedule. The longest run suggested was 20-22 miles. It suddenly dawned on me that it was a long way to run. I'd studied the course for months before the Great North and visualised running the half marathon, but this suddenly seemed even scarier than I could imagine. I was familiar with the map of London, but the idea of running this route seemed huge.

I'd got the buzz of running and wanted to keep it up, so the goal of doing the London Marathon kept my hunger for training runs going. My dad lived on the south coast and ran the Bournemouth Bay Half Marathon many years ago, and he suggested I look at doing the same. After a quick internet search, I found out it was in March. Ideal! That would fit into my training plan. A few friends had also done the Silverstone Half Marathon, which also fell in March, so that was scheduled into the regime.

I continued those little runs and fitted them in with my love of playing football. I use the term playing football loosely as my skill level in that sport hadn't improved much since my school days, but my confidence and passion had ramped up a few levels. I was running the Cobblers Fans Team. Being a huge supporter of Northampton Town Football Club, this would be the closest I would ever get to playing for the team I've supported since a kid. We would meet fellow opposition fans on match days and play a friendly match. It was brilliant! No real skill was needed, and the ethos was about having fun. This ticked so many boxes. My teammates, including Sid, who I ran the Silverstone 10K with, were very supportive of my London Marathon entry and were already asking for my sponsorship forms. Likewise with work colleagues, so I was now committed.

As the new year arrived, I started to increase my mileage and got ready for my second half marathon at Silverstone. The event was very different from the Great North and involved four different laps of the world-famous circuit. Although there wasn't the raucous support lining the course, it was a brilliant experience with around 5,000 runners snaking around the wide track. I finished in 1:49:59, almost ten minutes quicker than my first half. It was my first official new personal best (PB).

A few weeks later, I was excited to be running the Bournemouth Bay Run. After spending many childhood summers on Southbourne beach with my nan while visiting my dad, it's a place that's always been special to my heart. The route was mainly along the promenade, hugging the golden sands where I'd built many a sandcastle, ate ice creams and paddled in the sea. Jules and I also chose Bournemouth as the place for our wedding. We'd toyed with a Caribbean beach but settled for a low-key affair at the registry office in the popular seaside resort. It was beautiful, simple, casual, laid back and quiet. I wore a pair of combat trousers and smart trainers, which will probably not surprise many people who know me. Jules wore a beautiful blue designer dress. After getting married, we went for a Chinese meal and then played crazy golf in the Central Gardens with the handful of people we'd told. Some people go to Gretna Green for a secret wedding; we travelled to the opposite end of the country.

Anyway, back to the race! It was a pleasant spring morning with a calm breeze and blue skies. The route made its way from Bournemouth Pier along the promenade and up into Durley Chine, a beautiful tree lined pathway leading to the clifftop. After running along the road, we descended back to the sea, through Middle Chine, which was even more beautiful.

I got into a good rhythm, and my pace felt comfortable as I focused on Hengistbury Head, a lovely rocky area of natural beauty that jutted out into the sea in front of the Isle of Wight that sat behind it.

The emotion was tremendous as I passed the beach huts that we'd rent for our family holidays, and I could almost hear my nan's voice of encouragement in my head. She'd probably say something like, 'Running a half marathon, I dunno where you get your energy from boy!'

Nan always thought anything that required effort and dedication was an amazing feat and wondered how it could be done. After a loop of Southbourne, the route retraced itself to return to the finish line at Bournemouth Pier. I spotted Jules and my dad in the crowd as I quickened my pace to cross the finish line with another PB of 1:47 exactly.

Do you sometimes find that your love of one thing distracts you from focusing on another goal? I'd realised that I loved the half marathon distance and coupled with the buzz of playing football for fun, it was becoming hard to build up to that 20-mile training run. The longest I managed before the marathon day was 16.5 miles, which was an experience. It was in driving rain, hail, sleet, snow and sunshine. I also didn't take enough water and jumped into a shop a few miles from home to buy and down a bottle of a well-known orangey sports brand.

London Baby
The big day in April 2008 arrived, and Jules and I made our way to the capital to collect my number from the expo the day before. I was shaking with excitement. We were staying at my sister Katy's place, conveniently located in Woolwich, a short hop from the start.

If I can give any first-time marathoner advice, there would be quite a long list. Firstly, run further than 16.5 miles if you're planning to run the whole distance without taking a walk break. By the way, there's nothing wrong with walking in a marathon. Also, avoid a full day of sightseeing the day before your first big race. One more, eat more than a slice of toast for breakfast. Yep, I made all those mistakes but still loved my experience.

Arriving at Blackfriars, the pre-event buzz was huge. People were moving in many directions, but I plodded around, taking it all in. We made our way to the red start for charity runners. As we watched people lining up at the front, I planned to hop over the barrier and join the crowd. A marshal soon ended that idea and instructed me to enter from the back, which was a few minutes' walk. Suddenly, the race started, and I panicked; Jules and Katy gave me a quick pre-race hug and wished me good luck as I sprinted towards the back of the starting pen. After a few hundred metres, I realised I needn't run for two reasons. First, the race was 26.2 miles, and I needed to conserve energy. Secondly, it was chip timed, so it didn't matter if I was a couple of minutes late crossing the line.

Chip timing is excellent! If you're not familiar with the term, in running, it has nothing to do with how quickly you can eat a portion of a fried potato snack. Runners have an electronic microchip attached to their shoe or race number, and this activates as they cross a mat at the start line and then records an accurate race time when they cross another mat at the finish line. I've done some big events where it's taken me up to an hour to begin the race once the start gun has sounded. Please also note that not every race is actually started with a gun. This was something quite traditional. However, the *gun time* is sometimes also recorded at some events.

As I crossed the start line, it suddenly dawned on me that I was running the London Marathon. I called those words out loud, and the chap beside me replied, *"Me too mate!"*

Apologies to any residents from the Northeast who claim that the Great North Run is the best atmosphere in the world, but London was smashing it that day. Running through Woolwich's rough and ready suburbs with residents banging drums and playing loud music from speakers hanging out of their windows, the energy and noise were nothing like I'd heard before. Then came the Cutty Sark and the streets of Greenwich. I have goosebumps typing this, thinking of the incredible cheering crowd that was louder than any football match I've ever attended. It was impossible to run without gazing around to take it all in. I saw Jules and Katy waving energetically in the crowd and minutes later passed the YMCA charity bus, who were equally enthusiastic after spotting my running vest.

Tower Bridge soon arrived after a very wet section through Bermondsey. Again, the noise and support were something else. It was like a striker running in on goal to score in football but was relentless. When I reached the north side of the bridge, I wanted to turn around and run back.

A right turn at the Tower of London and the leading runners suddenly come back in the opposite direction. These guys were five or so miles ahead of us at this point. While watching them, I noticed a couple of football friends cheering in the crowd. The odds of seeing someone you know in the thousands of people are high so it is a big boost.

At 14 miles, ouch! My left knee suddenly felt a huge shooting pain below the knee cap. For a short moment, I felt sick. I didn't want to stop running now but was reduced to a quick walk. It felt awful as people were running past, and it didn't seem right to be walking in a marathon, although I've since learned that it's absolutely fine to do so. Thankfully, I managed to get going again and shake the pain off.

As mentioned, my longest training run was a very fragmented sixteen and a half miles in rain, sleet and snow. We'd already had rain and sleet but no snow on this day. I got to 17 miles around Canary Wharf and suddenly felt the energy drain from my body and mind. My legs just wanted to give up and stop. I staggered sideways and bumped into a couple of fellow runners who understood my apologies. Looking at a traffic island, I had the urge to sit down and stop for a rest.

The best thing about running through Canary Wharf on marathon day is that the noise bounces off the skyscrapers and amplifies it tenfold. This was exactly what I needed for a boost as my legs suddenly sprung back into life. An additional bonus was the sun breaking through the clouds adding a lovely effect, shining down from the mirrored glass buildings.

Rain, sleet and sunshine, what next? Yep, snow! That's right, in April, it snowed! Just what wasn't needed at the 19-mile marker. At this point, the opposite side of the road was open to traffic and the crowds weren't quite as busy as other parts of the course. It was time to really dig in and find strength. I resorted to a bit of walking followed by running as far as I could, cursing the training runs I ditched in favour of a football match.

I dragged myself to the Embankment alongside the River Thames, and the noise levels had regained good levels as the sun began to break through once again. The crowd knew that runners were in the last few miles, and the looks on some people's faces were that of sheer encouragement and awe of us on the roads.

'*Go on Groovy Grampa*' was a shout from some ladies I ran past. An elderly gentleman flew past me a moment later, leaving me in his wake. Seeing someone older looking so strong at this point was awe-inspiring, and something else which spurred me on.

Big Ben got closer, and so did the 25-mile sign. This wasn't a place to switch off as the boisterous support carried my every step. It felt easier than the first mile now, and I ran with a massive grin, high fiving as many people as possible. I continued along Birdcage Walk, around the corner towards Buckingham Palace and underneath a bridge that said, '385 yards to go', running past Buckingham Palace on my left and turned into The Mall to see the finish line.

Jules and Katy had kindly been given tickets to the VIP grandstands only 100 yards from the finish. By now, I was almost sprinting while trying to keep my excitement in check. I saw them both cheering and, trying to look casual, waved to them while covering those final steps. Arms aloft, I'd done it! I felt like a champ running through the finish arch before a volunteer put a medal around my neck. A lady beside me also shared the same delight, screaming, '*Oh my god, I've done it! I've done it; I've run the London Marathon!*'. She immediately burst into tears of joy and started hugging every stranger within a two-metre radius. She thanked me for some reason and continued her celebrations. It was a wonderful moment to experience the joy of a complete stranger who I'll probably never see again.

I found Jules and Katy in Horse Guards and sat on the grass in St James Park with the glorious sunshine blessing us. We swapped tales of running and spectating this fantastic event and realised how breath-taking and emotional it is seeing thousands of everyday people pushing themselves for many different reasons.

The next task was to find a pub where the YMCA crew were based for an after-race party. It wasn't too far away, and before long, I was sipping a complimentary pint and being handed snacks from a small buffet while receiving thanks from the charity's staff and volunteers. It was such a humbling experience, and their gratitude was heartfelt.

After another pub stop and food stop, we headed back to Waterloo Station to catch the train back to Woolwich, where the car was parked. I felt like a celebrity as the Transport for London staff opened each gate to let me onto the platform. One benefit of running the London Marathon is that competitors get free travel for the day of the event. You also get an amazing smile and congratulations and fellow travellers offering up seats to runners and congratulating people wearing medals. The togetherness of the London Marathon was unifying.

The following week, I felt the need to drop my marathon achievement into almost every conversation. That's if someone hadn't mentioned it first. The most asked question was, *'What was your time?'* I was delighted with 4:56:47. The second most common question was, *'Are you going to do it again next year?'* My answer was yes. Many people also made an age-old joke that they'd rather have a Snickers than a marathon. Yep, Snickers chocolate bars used to be called Marathon many years ago and, if you ever do a marathon, I guarantee a non-running friend will make that wise crack.

I reached my fundraising target of over £1,300 for YMCA and had several phone calls from them afterwards. The area director called to thank me personally, and I was also featured in their quarterly magazine. A personalised, handwritten thank you card arrived in the post; the love and appreciation made it even more worthwhile. That was it - I was now officially a marathon runner!

————

Stories From the Field - Real Life Marathon Runners

Jodie's Marathon

I caught up with my friend Jodie, who now lives in the Canary Islands. Shortly before she moved out, she completed the London Marathon. She told me her story,

'What on earth was I thinking? I was so inspired by my incredible running club buddies that I impulsively entered the 2013 London Marathon ballot. I didn't tell anyone as I felt a bit embarrassed to think I was actually capable of such a thing; marathons were events that faster, fitter, and exceptional people did. At that point I'd only been running for five months and not more than a 10K.

When I received a place through the ballot, I had mixed feelings: excited, overwhelmed, and embarrassed that, for the countless running friends who'd received another rejection after years of trying, this just wasn't fair!

Over the winter months, the hard miles in early mornings, cold, wet, wind, ice and snow clocked up. I loved (most) of those runs and races, with good friends and wonderful people. We each had our goals and challenges, and I hope those times were mutually supportive and beneficial to everyone.

Marathon day arrived and it was too hot for running. The idea of running 26.2 miles in anything other than cold, snow, sleet, rain and low temperatures filled me with dread. I was not at all prepared for it.

After finding the bag drop, the toilets and the water supply, I met up with a few of my club runners who were amazingly calm, which was reassuring. I was in pen nine, based on an estimated time, you are placed with runners of a similar pace. I drifted further to the back of that group, knowing I didn't want to be tempted into running faster than my usual pace.

Unceremoniously, people started moving forward, and the race appeared to have started. Half a mile from the start line, I drifted along with the thousands of others who were planning on walking/running. Some were dressed up as sharks, rhinos or even teacups.

And then, there it was - the start of the marathon. Hundreds of people by the side of the road screaming, cheering, shouting, clapping, calling out people's names, blowing whistles, banging drums, bands, music... and on and on for the best part of 26.2 miles. I've never known anything like it. The supporters were phenomenal, the noise deafening, and the atmosphere was like a carnival. Up until about 22 miles the streets were lined with hundreds of people in excellent spirits, giving food, drinks and support along the way. There were no sarcastic comments, jeers or anything other than a party-like atmosphere. Everyone wanted to slap my hand! The first five miles flew by... but then the cramps started.

I'd never experienced cramps like this before. The feeling of being stabbed in my calf just stopped me in my tracks. I stopped to rub some gel on it, stretch and try running again. This went on for the next ten miles... running a couple of hundred metres, then these sharp stabbing cramps in one, or both of my calves, then starting in my thighs. This was disastrous!

To make matters worse, after 13 miles, I stopped at a corner where a few St. John Ambulance volunteers were offering big daubs of Vaseline. I made the fatal error of taking my shoe off as the blisters were becoming uncomfortable by then. I had a walnut-sized blister on the inside of my right foot, where I'd always got blisters. No wonder it bloody hurt! I smeared Vaseline over my foot, a token plaster, sock and trainer on, and continued.

I ran on and off for another couple of miles before the cramp in my calves was too horrific to continue. Around 15 miles, I resigned myself to getting nowhere near the six-hour time I was hoping for and then faced with walking the remaining 11 miles and the challenge of getting in before the eight-hour cut-off point.

It would have been easy to quit. People all around me were dropping out or being treated by St. John's, but I was no more injured than when I started. I had the energy and stamina in my legs but just couldn't run on them because of the cramps and blisters. So, I marched on...I kept trying to work out what my walking pace would have to be to get in before eight hours.

Whilst the atmosphere continued to be incredible, I was overtaken by several Rhinos, a giant Peppa Pig, a teacup, a shark and a surfboard. I was also growing a little tired of Annie, a lady dressed entirely in red, who bounced, skipped and danced for the crowd. She stopped every 100 yards and played four bars of the song 'Bring Me Sunshine' on the red trumpet. She loved it, and the crowd loved it, but for me and a few other dozen people all going at the same pace, it was pretty irritating after eight miles of it. I wanted to shove it down her throat, bless her! I stopped for a toilet break just to lose her, I think.

I recommend taking toilet tissue on any long run, particularly a marathon! The first toilet cubicles were clean and well stocked with loo-roll, but at 13 and 18 miles, having been used by hundreds of hot, sweaty, dehydrated, loose-bowelled runners, you can guarantee that a foul-smelling faeces-smeared toilet cubicle is the last place you want to get your butt out! There would be more dignity and hygiene in 'doing a Paula Radcliffe' and squatting at the side of the road. Human waste is quite unpleasant!

At 18 miles, the pain from the blisters was excruciating. It felt like walking on fire. Moist, where the showers and sweat had soaked into my shoes, it felt like my feet were bleeding and squelching between my toes. Then I just cried... pretty much constantly for the remaining eight miles. I've never known pain like it (I'd rather go through labour again!) but having got that far there was just no way I could stop. I just had to shut down, block everything else out, and focus on powering through the pain.

I'd previously read that slower runners and walkers may have to make way for the sweeper tractors and clean-up crews, but this was awful. For the last few miles, the toughest of all, supporters had gone home, others were taking down the barriers, and the noise and dust created by the tractors, vans and buses were choking and demoralising.

Then I saw a lovely friend Neil at 25 miles. Knowing I only had a little way to go and having a final push and support from Neil was fantastic.

However, getting around the corner and seeing the finish line was anti-climactic at best. 'You've got to raise your arms and look happy,' the photographer shouted at me! I kept my thoughts to myself, grimaced and raised my arms as much as I could. Robotically handed a medal and chip timer removed. Marshals were exhausted too and barely able to give me any clear instructions about where my bag was. Broken, I hobbled for another mile to where they'd dumped all the late baggage. But I didn't care, I had my medal and wanted to find my husband Pete and daughter Lucy and flop on the grass; I was an emotional and physical wreck, but I got my medal.

Almost ten years on from her story, I asked Jodie if she'd ever do another marathon. She replied, 'Never Again! London? No. Never. However, anyone who thinks about a marathon I think should think about doing it. It's an incredible experience and the atmosphere is fantastic. I'm eternally grateful, humbled and inspired by people's friendships, support, dedication and encouragement.'

Sharky's Marathon

'I ran the London Marathon 2003 in a time of 4.45 and swore I would never run another marathon again. My abiding memory is that I was so hungry at the finish that I ate the pack of microwave Bolognese sauce and the pack of microwave pasta that was in the goodie bag. Both tasted awful, being cold and uncooked but down they went. I treasured the medal, which is still one of my favourites today.'

'Never again' is quite ironic as Sharky is a legend on the marathon scene and has clocked up almost 200 to date. He also inspired me to officially enter the 100 Half Marathon Club, but we'll talk more about that later in the book.

Paula's Marathon

I've known Paula for several years but didn't know the story of her first run. 'I have so many running memories, but my favourite was in 2012 when I ran the London Marathon. Having sat and watched the race on the TV for years and never thought that I was capable of running at all, let alone 26.2 miles. I entered the ballot and got in! My aim was to run it in less than five hours. With 25 minutes to get in on target, I had a mile and a half to go so I decided to lap up the atmosphere and run-walk the last bit as I didn't think I would ever run the London Marathon again; I felt like a celebrity, when I crossed the finish line, I felt so proud of myself and overcome with emotion. My finish time was 4.59.58!'

Daniel's Marathon

Daniel is a local runner who is pretty quick on the track. We caught up after a parkrun recently and he told me his marathon story:

'I have run one marathon as it was always on the bucket list. After securing a charity place, I had just over four months to train. Halfway into training, I fell off my bike on the way to work. The chain slipped, and I went down onto the bike handlebars and had to be checked out at A&E. However, the pain was just the ribs being badly bruised, leaving me underprepared. At that point, the furthest I'd run was fourteen miles, so I had no idea what to expect.

I'd managed to raise a few thousand pounds in a short time, so all was set. I was around nineteen miles in when I regretted not getting more long runs in, hitting the wall (yes, not a brick wall). I had seven more miles of walk/jog to come and certainly appreciated the handing out of bananas and jelly babies from the crowd from that point onwards.

It's strange how your body just shuts down and movement becomes limited. I now understand why there are half marathons and marathons.

I never uttered the words never again. However, I said I needed to train more and slow down in the first half. The clear evidence was that there just was not enough power in the legs for breaking four hours. I meandered across the line in four hours 42 minutes, which is strange as my half PB is one hour 36 minutes.

It was great to see London lined with people cheering your name. A tip is to get your name on your t-shirt. People cheering for you is a welcome motivation, strangely.

The greatest reason I did the marathon, however, was to show my children what I could achieve, and they would also be able to achieve their goals of doing a marathon and wasn't out of reach for them.'

Darren's Marathon

'The first marathon I entered was the London Marathon in 2007 through the open ballot in which I raised money for cleft lip and palate (CLAPA). I was overwhelmed by the whole experience and the day's atmosphere. Runners from all parts of the world are running for their chosen charities to make a big difference. I will never forget the energy in the spectators lining the streets of London, encouraging all runners to keep going. This really motivated me, especially around the 20-mile mark when your legs are heavy and you feel like giving up. Still, somehow you seem to find the extra inner strength from somewhere to push yourself through the pain, totally focused on why you are running a marathon in the first place. Reaching the last 400 metres, I had so many mixed emotions tearful, joyful, relief and suddenly the shock you've just crossed the finish line and received that all-important medal for which you've trained so hard. What an achievement. My first marathon time was four hours and two minutes!'*

Darren is a new running friend who I met during the pandemic. A fellow runner put out an appeal to help a blind runner complete a virtual marathon in less than four hours. That was a little too quick for me, so I reached out on our running club's social media page, and John, offered to help. To cut a long story short, they did it. Darren and John have become really good mates now, and Darren trusts in John to guide him around the obstacles he can't see. Darren is also an open-water swimmer and cyclist, showing that obstacles can be overcome. Most of all, it shows the wonderful community spirit found in running. We'll hear more from Darren later.

David's Marathon

I thought I'd finish with a short and sweet anecdote from David, who shared, *'It was my one and only marathon, Nottingham 2014. It felt like I'd died and gone to another place! That's what happens when you don't train as well as you should have. Honestly, though, lots of emotions. Pride, wondering why I hurt in places I didn't know existed and just wanting to go to sleep. That medal is an important milestone I'll always look back on.'*

———

Thoughts Running Through the Mind

This book is about the story of my half marathon journey, but you can't write half marathon without the word marathon.

I've found that I can run a half and feel comfortable, but a full marathon takes my body to a place where it's not entirely happy. You can see this from my running friend's stories above too. The words *outside your comfort zone* can be overused in life, but they are true of achieving success. Magic generally happens when you are brave and daring.

Now, you don't have to run a marathon, but life goals are typically long-haul events. When we took our first flight to Southeast Asia, it took twelve hours to get there. That's a long time to spend on a plane but it was necessary to reach the destination.

Think about a big goal you'd like to achieve in your life and the steps involved. A marathon isn't 26.2 miles! It's deciding to enter it and then putting together a training plan. It could be running the first run to the end of the road and having to get in shape before going much further. It's the consistent training runs and building up the distance over the weeks and months leading up to the event. It's buying the right kit, eating the right food and making the travel plans the day before. All those steps have to happen before the 26.2 miles take place.

In the chapter, Crossing the Line, I challenged you to set a goal to do something new. This time, think of a big, audacious goal. A marathon sized one. Be brave and write it down and then you can start planning your steps to achieve it later.

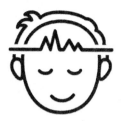

6. Carefree Running

After the London Marathon, running became even more integrated into my life. I found myself juggling activities between that, football and gym sessions. I sometimes couldn't choose between a race and a football match, so I'd do both on some weekends. Before watching the main game in the afternoon, it would be off to some random place to play for the Northampton Town Fans Team. Home, sleep and then up for a 10K or half marathon the following day.

One weekend, I played football in Barnet, North London against a side that fielded some youth team footballers. It was against the spirit of fans team football, and we got run ragged all over the pitch. We had no substitutes, so it meant a full 90 minutes. The temperature hit 28 degrees that day to make things harder, which was bizarre for the first weekend in October. After dashing to the ground and seeing Northampton win (which was rare at Barnet), we drove home. The following day, I ran a PB at the Northampton 10K, which fittingly started and finished at Sixfields Stadium, home of Northampton Town Football Club. The weather was just as hot.

My running times were falling, and I was getting personal bests at all distances. I'd also joined Northampton Road Runners and realised running clubs are not cliquey. This was the best decision I've made in my running career, and I have been a member ever since.

I went back and ran the Great North Run and London the following year. The Great North seemed much busier but still had a great atmosphere. I ran London for another charity, but they weren't quite as friendly as YMCA. Both were brilliant, but I found all sorts of different events through friends at my running club.

The big events were amazing. Doing the very first London 10,000 was pretty special. It was nice to run a 10K around the capital's sights without having to hit the wall of the marathon. On this particular day, it hammered down with rain, and as I made my way to the start in Birdcage Walk, near Buckingham Palace. A confused marshal let me into the starting area through the elite funnel. I hadn't realised I'd taken a wrong turn until a lady performing her pre-race drills ran straight into me. Breaking from her focus, she apologised profusely. I then realised it was Olympic marathon athlete Liz Yelling. Realising I was somewhere I probably shouldn't have been, I graciously accepted Liz's apology and walked through several other elite athletes before lining up as close to them as possible but not trying to stand out too much. When the race started, it was like seeing a row of cars driving off into the distance. However, the event was amazing as I was ahead of the mass crowds and enjoyed the race, finishing with a PB.

Aside from the big events, I did smaller local ones like the Wellingborough 5 mile, the Rugby 6 mile and the Milton Keynes 10K. I loved racing and enjoyed the push to a half marathon, participating in the Cransley Half, Bedford Harriers Half and Milton Keynes Half.

After not wanting the pressure of a specific fundraising target, I'd entered London through the ballot to have a third go but was unsuccessful, so a new challenge was needed. Instead of doing a marathon, I opted for four half marathons in four consecutive weeks and friends, family and work colleagues were impressed enough to donate to charity again. This time, it was for Help for Heroes. My line-up was the Milton Keynes Running Festival, Silverstone Half Marathon, Water of Life Half and a finish at the Bournemouth Bay Run.

It was such a buzz! I broke one hour and forty minutes for the first time at MK and decided to go for better at Silverstone. However, in the last few miles, my legs fell off (not literally), and I dropped my pace a little for a more comfortable finish. The Water of Life was my first real trail run experience, with some of the route alongside the Thames going out from Bisham Abbey. I loved it! Bournemouth was my special place, and I gave up on pushing for a PB to enjoy the event. After the run, Jules took a picture for my Fundraising page, and I wore all four finisher medals whilst standing on the beach. This also took me up to a total of 14 half marathon run in around two and a half years. The love affair was there for sure. From 5K to 10K to half marathon and some random distances between, I loved it. Road races, cross country, trail runs, I would have a go at all sorts of events.

I did the London Marathon twice more with Rutland Marathon sandwiched between but found a point where I just wanted to stop during the race, and, somehow, I couldn't seem to break my target of a sub-four-hour finish. In the Olympic year of 2012, I got close with a time of 4:06:04. I wasn't sure if playing football was perhaps getting in the way, but I was now following a training plan and doing the 20-mile Sunday runs, even in the rain and snow. One thing that helped was having like-minded friends to run with.

After my Lodnon 2012 effort being so close to that four hour barrier, I began to think about the following year. Would I take a break from football and go for it? Well, that choice was made for me.

Fate Works in Mysterious Ways

Sometimes, fate works in weird ways. In August that year, I had to accept that I'd kicked a football for the last time. My final 11-a-side match was at Sixfields Stadium, where our fans team played a charity match against Northampton Town's staff and some former players. We'd managed to arrange this as an end-of-season climax for the past three years, and it was special to play at the home of the club I'd supported all my life. Playing against players I'd watched from the stands for years was equally humbling. I'd even convinced Jules that we would book a shorter holiday to Majorca that week so I could make it home for the match. After a six-day trip, I was home and putting on my football kit to take to the hallowed turf. However, I was blissfully unaware until a few months later, that I would be pleased to have made this decision.

As I sat in a medical room of John Radcliffe Hospital three months later. I was told to avoid contact sports for at least six months, following that freak head injury on our next holiday in Fuerteventura. Those six months became another six months before being told, perhaps don't play again, the risk was too high. Getting the advice to stop doing something I loved was hard to process. The fans team was a big part of my life, it provided a safe place to play uncompetitive football and not worry about my lack of skill.

However, the specialist had countered my massive disappointment with the good news that I could go for a light jog. The swelling on my brain hadn't expanded, and it was expected to disperse over the next three to six months. Only a month before, I'd been cramming as much crazy and carefree stuff into our lives, and, after performing an everyday task, I was now lucky to be alive. It's not often that a trip to the toilet has such devastating consequences. OK, some of my friends may joke about using the bathroom after I've been there, but there was no toilet humour innuendo intended here, this was serious. A few weeks before, I'd smashed my PB at the Wellingborough Five Mile and felt ready to step up to the next level in my quest for running glory. I couldn't face stopping now, and this accident felt like it would get in the way of my life. I was scared, but there was no time for that; it was time to get back on track and do a test run. The local parkrun had recently begun at the park right opposite our house. If anything went wrong, there would be plenty of people around, and I was only a few minutes from home. Better still, we live a ten-minute walk from the hospital too.

It was fine. I started at the back and got around the course in a time that was only two minutes slower than my regular time. Perhaps this head injury wasn't as serious as I thought. Despite being urged by my loving family and friends to take it easy, I was desperate to return to being a carefree spirit again. I don't know if you've ever experienced a trauma where you go into denial? I was clearly in denial and began to play down the after-effects of my recovery period. Friends kept telling me I didn't look right, but I did my best to shrug it off and pretend I was OK. Our local club organised the Moulton 10K, and I agreed to help as usual. I had friends insisting I wasn't left alone, just in case I blacked out or felt funny. Deep down inside, I was so grateful for these offers as I found it difficult to focus.

Things didn't add up. One minute, I was running a PB. Next, I was on holiday and enjoying a lovely meal, and then I was laid up in a hospital bed, hearing that people don't survive that level of a blow to the head. Perhaps if I'd been participating in some form of dangerous extreme sports, I'd have been able to understand what had happened. However, all I'd done was go to the toilet. When some people sustain an injury doing something, they can sometimes be nervous about doing that task again. Unfortunately, I had to get back in the saddle (so to speak) on that one as it was unavoidable not making a trip to the bog again.

These feelings circulated in my mind: cheated, in denial, dismissive, scared, sad, ecstatic, and invincible.

Running-wise, I stuck to my local parkrun. Now parkrun is the best thing ever. That's probably the world's biggest exaggeration for some people, but it arrived in Northampton and exploded with a bang. On the tenth anniversary of the start of the Northampton parkrun, there were nine in the county alone and talk of a tenth. That's not to mention the hundreds more in villages, towns and cities all over the country. Despite the confident facade I was putting on, my inner self was still terrified and confused, and parkrun provided that safe space to run.

Then came the next blow! Six weeks after my head injury, I was stunned as my beautiful, kind-hearted and caring mother-in-law suddenly passed away. Just like that! She departed this planet without warning or sign and left Jules, me, and our family heartbroken. She came to our house for a Sunday get-together in celebration of my mum's birthday, and when she left, her last words to me were '*Be careful and take a bit more care.*'

With my brain suffering from the damage, I couldn't process what had happened. I wanted to cry but couldn't. Grief wouldn't come as I felt empty. I was trying to recover from the confusion and fogginess in my head, but now there was an external blow to deal with. I just wanted to forget about my accident and be there for Jules and the rest of the family, but a fuzzy thought process would usually end in complete fatigue, and I'd need to go and lie down. Jules handed in her notice at work, gave up a demanding job, and decided to join me in our business. At the time, I was a freelance presenter, delivering motivational training seminars to schools all around the country, and we also had a network marketing business. It made sense to work on this together. We pushed on to the end of the year, and finally, after Christmas, Jules left her job.

We're a solid couple but had been dealt a double blow. I was still driving long distances and struggled to shake this foggy feeling and focus. However, I needed to move on from this and put it down to the healing process. And, running provided a big release for me. I needed a new focus, so I entered the Paris Marathon. Jules was behind me on this and thought it would be good to have a focus and a break.

My training began in January, and I started to enter races to get used to running more than a few miles. First the Irchester 15K Dirt Run, then the Charnwood Hills Fell Race and the Belvoir Challenge, half-marathons number 29 and 30. The next one followed at Berkhamsted, followed by a couple of 20-mile races and then onto Paris.

Three weeks after Paris, I found myself running the Shakespeare Marathon. OK, it wasn't just by chance, as that might have sounded. I missed that elusive sub-four-hour barrier in the French capital and thought, what the hell, I've trained for a marathon, so let's do another. I did 4:03:41 at Paris and was eight seconds slower at Stratford. However, there was no disappointment. If I could run a marathon after a life-threatening injury, I could achieve anything. Despite the fogginess, forgetfulness and the fatigue, I was back.

In the Shakespeare Marathon, the first couple of miles of the route looped around the town centre of Stratford twice, taking in the beautiful old buildings and past the birthplace of Shakespeare himself. Passing along a narrow street busy with runners, my mate and I hopped onto the pavement to skirt around a car that a resident hadn't removed. A marshal greeted us with an angry fist, shouting, 'Get back on the road; this is a road race, not a bloody pavement race!'

It was met with howls of laughter from all the runners in earshot, and the Victor Meldrew-like character continued his angry first waving at anyone else who dared to venture across the threshold of the gutter. No disrespect to the elderly marshal, who was doing an excellent job, but simple moments like that stick in the memory and bring a smile.

After completing my seventh marathons, I felt physically fit and was in great running form. A couple of weeks later, I ran my fastest 10K at Silverstone, back where it all began. However, this epic training journey for Paris and Stratford may have left me in good physical shape, but mentally I was drained. That brain fog felt a little heavier between the moments of joy and exhilaration. I decided it was time to go back to what I loved, the half marathon. The beautiful 13.1 miles seemed appealing, and I knew I had to slow down my pace a little, so I entered some events that required off-road sections. A few low-key races that were favourites with our club were the Otmoor Challenge, a glorious countryside route that started and finished at a village fair on a Saturday afternoon.

There was also the Adderbury Half which was another rural route in Oxfordshire. The appealing thing was the route seemed to change each year due to unforeseen circumstances. The first time I did this event, the course had flooded the night before thanks to unseasonable July rain. With just over a mile to go, I noticed a marshal standing by a stile that we had to hop over. He warned me to be careful on the bridge with a massive grin on his face. As I navigated the stile, I noticed the bridge was a foot underwater from the flood, which meant wading across the stream, cleaning the mud off my shoes in the process. All great fun!

In the latest running of this race, temperatures hit 30 degrees as we finished. It was energy sapping, and, for some reason, the course was a mile longer this year. My watch clocked 14.1 miles as I crossed the line. A few of our running club drove to Birmingham afterwards to watch an athletics meeting, and the commentator asked spectators to shout out to the 400-metre runners who had to run in such high temperatures. We sat back and tutted in jest. All they had to do just one lap of a track, we'd just done over 14 miles across tought terrain.

A special race arrived in September when Jules and I travelled to Dorset for The Beast. This was the race I'd entered the previous year, and when the medical team at John Radcliffe Hospital advised me to live my life as normal, I excitedly announced that I'd entered The Beast. Hopes of running it were soon quashed, the specialist saying that normal people don't run races called The Beast. Here is a description of the race on the organisers' website: 'The Beast is just that, a beast of a race. Taking in some of the most spectacular views of Dorset (well, in our humble opinion), the 13(ish) mile 'undulating' course starts on Corfe Castle Common before heading out towards Worth Matravers and then on to the coastal path with great views of the sea! The course then heads back towards Corfe with only a few 'minor' hills to get up.'

After being told that I shouldn't run the event, I emailed the organisers, explained my head injury and asked if I could defer my place a year. I told them that it would be amazing to be able to recover to take part a year later. Some independent events like this may say no, but The Beast kindly said they would give me free entry for 2013. So, it became my goal to run this event.

Jules and I stayed in Bournemouth for the weekend. We enjoyed the Bournemouth Air Festival, which, as you'd expect for the last weekend in August, was busy, noisy and over-stimulating, something that brain injury struggles with. I didn't care, though; I was in one of my happy places again and dismissing any signals my mind was trying to send to me.

Race day was emotional in many ways. I'd arranged to meet my dad at Corfe Castle before the start, but he couldn't find us. There was a crowd of runners next to a bloody great big castle, and we somehow missed each other. As I crossed the start line, I had tears in my eyes as it was a year on from that trauma to the head. OK, I'd done a couple of marathons and other events, but this was the one I'd eyed up as a pinnacle in my recovery. It must've seemed strange to the small crowd of spectators to see a runner crying within the first hundred metres of a race that's not for the faint-hearted. After a loop down a hill and back up again, I went past Jules, stopped for an emotional hug, and then headed out into some stunning countryside, going up and down some more hills. Suddenly the world opened up to a view over the English Channel from the top of the Jurassic cliffs where the route hugged a coastal path. There were a few more tears of emotion at the immense, raw beauty that unfolded. A few feet to the left was a sheer drop into the sea. I felt fragile as my life was endangered by going to the toilet, and this required a bit of focus, although the path was safe. The trail then dropped to sea level and climbed a cliff of around 150 feet on the other side. It was immense!

I crossed the line and shed more tears. This race felt so special, and for the first time in ages, I'd been able to cry. Perhaps this was the release I needed. Jules was waiting with a huge hug. As we turned to walk away, I heard a guy call out, *It's Mark, isn't it?* Turning around, a man stood with his hand stretched out for a handshake. Instinctively I grabbed his palm with a curious look. *'I've been looking out for you and wanted to say welcome to The Beast and congratulations on completing it. Wow, you've been through so much with your head injury!'* It was the race organiser and he'd seen me cross the line shortly before. It's moments like these when you realise how wonderful people really are. Sometimes, a simple comment or a smile to a stranger can have the biggest impact on the recipient.

Half marathon number 35 had been completed, and it was part of an emotional weekend that was to get more emotional. Jules and I left the event and headed to Swanage for some lunch. We'd shared some nice trips there with my late mother-in-law, whose passing was still very raw almost a year on. As we stood, looking over the sea before heading home, we took a moment to reflect on a lovely weekend and how important happiness and love are in life.

Perhaps this release had been a good thing, and I could go back to being that carefree runner I was just over a year ago. Sadly, it wasn't to be. Half marathon number 36 was that fateful September day when the band Madness came to Northampton.

———

45

Stories From the Field - Real Life Runners Finishing

It van be really hard to pull yourself out of a dark place and get back on track. This can happen in life, but the running route can sometimes throw up some negative thoughts and challenge your own belief and sanity. However, when you get to the finish line, that negativity can disappear and turn into tears of joy and elation.

Pete shared his story. *'I was doing my first ultra, and from the 20-mile mark, I kept doubting my ability to finish, but thanks to a running buddy, we got it done. After crossing the finish line, the doubt, tiredness and aches disappeared briefly. Even now, I think about it, and it's still sinking in.'*

Mark said, *'I was running the 70-mile Rat Race, The Wall. There were many dark moments as we ran into the night but crossing that line with my friend Paul and having our support crew at the finish line was unbelievable. It made me cry tears of joy and pain!'*

Sue had to stop running after a foot operation but has thankfully returned to what she loves. *'At the St Neots Half, I knew I shouldn't have run as my foot was not fully healed. I cried for the first three miles but then had a serious talk to myself. When I finished, I cried but felt the need to do that run again pain-free. I'm told it's a lovely course, but I can't remember it!'*

Richard also kindly added, *'It's all good to be emotional. I did a race last weekend and had to dig deep to finish. I cried at the end, but it felt normal, and I didn't feel ashamed.'*

Rob recently recorded a brilliant PB at the Manchester Marathon, *'This year, I crossed the line at Manchester in 3:16 knowing I'd smashed my PB, while being physically and mentally broken. The happiness afterwards eating and drinking with my running buddies at the pub, plus catching up with a very old friend. Memories that will last a lifetime.'*

Chloe also had a tale from Manchester, *'My most emotional time running was the Manchester Marathon! I cried several times during the race: at halfway my headphones stopped working, then at 16 miles, I was sick. At 19 miles got a cramp down one leg and limped for a mile before hitting the wall at 22 miles. Then a friend caught me and ran with me to the end as I felt like I was going to die (a little bit of an overreaction, obviously). My finish time wasn't what I wanted, but I finished it!'*

Thoughts Running Through the Mind

Random acts of kindness are huge! Sometimes we underestimate how far a simple gesture can go. A great example above is runners supporting each other to get to the finish line. The organisers of The Beast also gave me such a wonderful feeling and a boost of confidence in my recovery.

Event organisers of small races have a big job on their hands, and it would've been easy for Poole Athletics Club to reply and say that they don't defer races and to make me pay again. Although I had picked up my running again since my head injury, this race became a milestone in my life. The comments from the race director at the end are probably stored away in a dusty filing cabinet in his memory banks now, but I won't forget that gesture.

On one of our holidays to the Canary Islands, I helped a retired couple carry their cases up three flights of stairs when we'd all checked into our hotel after a late arrival. As they thanked me, they reminded me that I'd also lifted their hand luggage into the overhead locker on the flight. That simple connection has led to a friendship with this lovely couple, who we have met on another holiday since, and we chat with them regularly.

Think about what random acts of kindness you could display to a stranger or even someone you know well. How could you carry out a simple act that would be well received?

Think about being kind to yourself too. In this busy world, we forget to take time out and stop for a moment. A friend of mine, a busy single mum with a stressful career, told me that it's selfish to go to a spa day with friends so she stayed home and missed out. Her life is sometimes at breaking point, she can be susceptible to illness and bugs but never stops because the kids need her, or she doesn't want to let her work colleagues down. It wouldn't be selfish for her to stop and have that deserved spa day. Her kids would be very supportive, and her ex-partner would welcome the extra day with his children. By practicing self-care, she would feel more relaxed and be able to build up her immune system to protect herself and her family and help to prevent her from being poorly.

It's sometimes easier said than done but think of ideas on how you could take time to relax and switch off. What's your favourite pastime that you've perhaps neglected and would be simple to do? Maybe there is something you could begin that could give you some *you time* or perhaps something that your family could also be involved in!

It's OK to ask for support and open up if you're struggling. It's OK not to be OK sometimes, and we should avoid being a superhero. Take time for yourself. Self-care is not selfish.

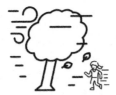

7. Running Into the Wind

There is something invigorating about jogging through a beautiful forest with the trees sheltering the summer sunshine or the mist hugging the green fields of the British countryside. I love this tranquillity of running as much as I love pounding my feet alongside the coast while listening to the crashing of the waves onto the beach.

I fondly remember my first experience of cross country. I am talking about my adult life, long since those days of being thrashed around the school field by my upper school PE teachers, who were less sympathetic than the excellent Mr. O'Neill at middle school.

As a relatively new member of my running club, I was soon roped into running for the cross-country team. Roped in is a pretty unfair description as I jumped at the chance to give it a go. It cost £3 to enter, and there was cake at the end. Yes, you had me at cake!

We all boarded a minibus and drove a short distance to a small village called Wing in Hertfordshire. After a short walk to the start line, the race began in the middle of a field. To coincide with the race start, the rain also began to fall. This was not part of the plans, of course.

The route was a lap around a field before making a sharp left turn and crossing an ankle-deep stream before heading further into the countryside. As the race progressed, the rain got harder and harder, and soon it was a mud fest underfoot. However, I loved this new challenge of running and trying to stay on my feet while going up or down a hill. The piece de resistance was the final crossing of the stream again before a sprint to the finish. Now, I forgot to mention there was a massive herd of cows in the field opposite the stream. They'd all happily hung around on the water's edge as we'd passed them 30 or so minutes beforehand. A combination of rain and cow poo had made its way into the water system that we now had to wade through in the last few hundred metres. Needless to say, the organisers insisted we remove our dirty shoes before heading inside the race HQ to dry off.

OK, so I may have loved this challenge, and there have been many other wet and muddy races that have been right up my street (although I guess it was a case of running along trails as opposed to streets). One thing I really struggle with is running into a headwind. If you add in cold rain, then I'm definitely not happy.

Lodes of Running and Grizzly Drizzle

My half marathon number 38 was in a small Cambridgeshire village called Lode. I learned about the race at the very last minute and got a lift there with my friend Charlotte. Much to our amusement, the organisers asked her if she was male or female when she registered. This question was also asked to my other friend Jim and then to me when we followed in the queue.

The Lode Half Marathon route was an out and back and went smoothly for the first six and a half miles. The turning point arrived, and we simply turned 180 degrees at a cone and retraced our steps. It was at that point that I realised that there was a near gale-force wind that had been behind us. I definitely swore more on the return leg and it took me around ten minutes longer.

Another fantastic event that wacky runners must do is The Grizzly. It's a 20ish-mile route on the south coast, starting in the Devon seaside town of Seaton. The whole town comes alive for Grizfest, with the race starting on a Sunday morning in early March.

After a mile-long stretch along a shingle beach, suddenly, we were climbing to the clifftops to enjoy the views from the top. It's one of the most random and fun events I've ever done (if you can call running 20 miles fun). One minute you're in a forest, and suddenly, you turn a corner and there's a guy playing the didgeridoo. Along the route are amusing motivational quotes to keep you smiling while pushing over some tough terrain. There are emotional shrines where you can pause for a moment and tie a ribbon to a teepee made from sticks and branches. Somewhere in the middle of the race is the bog of doom which consists of the stickiest mud I've ever encountered. It's about knee deep, and the only way to navigate your way through it is to lift your feet up to about waist height to free them from the bog. There's pretty much no escape from the gruelling slog through it. At the exit of the bog is a pile of shoes that the marshals claim to have pulled out of the bog.

I'd done the Grizzly twice before and loved it. The first time was unseasonably good weather with temperatures of around 15-16 degrees. There hadn't been much rain, so the ground was firm underfoot. The second time was the opposite. It had rained constantly throughout the month before the event and was as muddy as hell but great fun all the same. The third time was like the second but colder, wetter and icy at the start. As we lined up on the start line, the town crier prepared to give his usual address, but runners weren't really in the mood that year. We just wanted to get on our way as the temperature was just below freezing, with the bitter cold wind blowing in off the sea.

After the climb to the top of the cliffs, the wind was behind us, but it was open and very cold. The Grizzly was going to be a tough cookie this time. However, at the midway point, the course turned into a forest on a hillside and followed a beautiful woodland trail that snaked downwards into a valley. At this very point, giant snowflakes started to fall and settle on the trees around us. It was magical! When I reached the bottom of the valley, it looked like a winter wonderland postcard.

Ouch! Suddenly I had a shooting pain in my foot! As I was running through a muddy puddle, my heel struck a rock sticking out of the ground and it hurt like hell. A few steps later and I had to stop momentarily. Thankfully I managed to get going again, but the pain was evident and started to impact on my enjoyment of this event. It was now cold, wet sleet was falling from the sky, and my foot wasn't happy. The bog of doom was a welcome respite this year. Sheltered at the bottom of a crevice, walking through the soft and sticky mud was a relief to cushion my heel.

The final three miles were horrendous! The route turned onto the shingle beach at Branscombe, and I was battling a strong headwind with the sleet belting off the sea into my face. For good measure, there was the occasional hailstone. My gloves were soaking wet, and I decided to take them off as my hands were now colder than ever. I pulled my hat over my eyes and stared at the pebbles on the beach as I walked, swearing at every step. After a mile of run and walk, and trust me, there was more walking along the beach, we then made our way up the 'Stairway to Heaven', a steep cliff climb. Once at the top, and after more swearing, my legs had pretty much given up due to the cold. I couldn't feel my hands at all. It was time to dig deep and get to the end. A few fellow club members passed me, stopping to see if I was OK, but I urged them to continue. The final stretch into Seaton was downhill, and I hobbled over the line like a wounded war hero, cheered on by my club mates, who'd all waited the horrendous weather.

In the finish area, the fire service is armed with a hose to clean the mud off your trainers and legs, but I was in no mood for this. I was slightly worried that I couldn't now put any weight on my foot, so I went to the medical room. After a quick examination, the kind paramedic advised me that it was a slight bruise, but the pain was aggravated by the cold. I couldn't take my shoes off because my hands were bent into claws, so Jules had the not-so-lovely job of removing my muddy trainers.

An hour and a half later, I was changed and had returned to the pub a few metres from the finish line. The rain was lashing against the windows as the final finisher crossed the line. We did not envy the marshals and runners still out there as the weather worsened.

The numbness in my hands lasted for months. Despite the discomfort this caused, it never affected my love of running. These things can be part and parcel of the highs and lows, and I just found ways of preventing the numbness from returning. Friends have suggested doing muddy obstacle events which involve swimming in open water. This would be far too cold for my hands, plus risky to my head injury, having to climb over and crawl through things.

After the Grizzly, I went back to running half marathons. I did two more the following month: one was a multi-lap trail event in Northampton and then Stratford followed a week later. It was much nicer doing one lap of the course instead of the two for the previous year's Shakespeare Marathon. This took my half marathon total up to 43, and I'd set my goal to reach 50 by the end of the year.

Taking the Wind Out of My Sails
Now, I started this chapter talking about running into the wind. It was challenging, and my life had already taken a few blows with my head injury and the loss of my lovely mother-in-law, but suddenly, the wind was about to be taken out of my sails again. While travelling around the country to schools, I came home one Friday night from Manchester in the busy month of March. That day, I'd delivered a goal-setting programme at a school in Sale and had learnt that Cristiano Ronaldo had studied English there when he first moved to England and signed for Manchester United. When I slumped onto the sofa to tell Jules all the news, she stopped me in my tracks to tell me that she'd found a lump on her breast and was very worried. We wrote much more about this in our book *What The Hell Just Happened?*. After some scans and a few weeks of waiting, we were told the devastating news that it was breast cancer.

Not only did my hands feel numb, but I felt numb! I struggled to cope with my brain injury. The grief was still raw from the loss of my mother-in-law; now and my wife had been diagnosed with this. Our lives fell through the floor again! Jules faced a series of operations followed by lengthy treatment. The early news was very positive as the medical team assured us the tumour was tiny and contained, so it hadn't spread. However, life suddenly became harder than running into that gale force wind at the Lode Half Marathon and more numbing than the cold at the Grizzly.

Having done a lot of research into cancer, it's normal for the disease to attack someone vulnerable after experiencing traumas. Jules had lost her mum and almost her husband in a couple of months, so it became clear that this could've had a significant impact.

We tried to carry on with life in the most positive manner possible. Running was still my escape from the challenges life was throwing at us. Jules had her first operation when I ran my 44th half at the Milton Keynes Marathon Festival. I felt strong on the day and decided to run the event in my Northampton Town football shirt, hoping to get some banter from the rival Milton Keynes Dons football fans around the route. Still, I was more heartened to hear encouraging comments from Northampton fans who lived in MK or were visiting for the day.

MK is a relatively flat and winding course and the venue of a previous PB albeit on a different course. On this occasion, I felt strong and crossed the line in 1:36:59, a few minutes slower than before. I was pleased with my time, but as I walked through the stadium, I suddenly felt colossal panic washing over me. MK is less than 20 miles from Northampton, but I'd decided to go to the event on my own. I suddenly felt very alone and scared, knowing we faced such challenging months ahead. I sat in a corridor on the way out of the stadium and stared at the opposite wall. Fellow runners and their supporters were rushing past, full of smiles and joy at completing the event. My joy of a decent run was short-lived; it faded into the background.

Life was now beginning to blur. I was racing up and down the motorway (not literally, I'm a cautious driver) and visiting schools, coming home and being hit by fatigue from my brain injury. Jules was taking operations and preparation for treatment in her stride, but it was just surreal.

I did the Moulton Fun Run, a local village event a week after Milton Keynes. I led the race until the top of the highest point of the course, which gave me the annual award known as King of the Hill. Another runner caught me on the descent of the hill and beat me to the line, denying me a first-place finish. After receiving my King of the Hill award, I saw an old friend who asked me how Jules was. He didn't know about the cancer diagnosis, and I couldn't find the words to tell him.

At times, I just felt zapped of energy. It felt like I was running into a headwind all the time. Even on a beautiful June summer's day, I may as well have been running in those Grizzly-like conditions.

The Otmoor Challenge is on my favourites list. I've mentioned it before! It starts and finishes at a lovely village fair where everyone comes out in force. The first six miles are along farm tracks and country roads. It's beautiful and relatively quick. I was keeping a good pace in the hot summer sunshine and past the halfway point. Looking at my watch, I knew I was on for a good time. Then suddenly, something pulled a trigger, and it was as if the floor opened and swallowed me. I happened to notice a fellow runner was wearing a cancer charity t-shirt with a tribute to someone on it. Bang! It was as if a shot had been fired! Suddenly, my mind raced back to Jules's treatment and what she was about to undergo.

The cancer tumour had been removed in a mastectomy operation, but chemotherapy treatment was suggested to prevent any stray cancer cells from spreading. It was great news, but it was just scary. Jules was fit, active and healthy, but she was about to begin something which would make her very ill, and I was struggling to deal with that.

Seven miles into the Otmoor Challenge and I felt sick. Every time I broke into a jog, my stomach churned, and my head started to spin. By this point, the route had gone off-road and followed bridleways and trails around fields in the beautiful countryside. I began to walk, but that didn't feel great either. Fellow runners were passing and asking if I was OK. It's wonderful how many people break their running pace to stop and check in on someone else. As bizarre as it sounded, I just wanted to be alone. Do you ever have moments when you want to escape even the helping hands of well-wishers and supporters? It felt like a spotlight was shining on me in the middle of this field in Oxfordshire. It was far from civilisation with a few hundred or so runners, but I felt like I was on a national stage. My only choices were to hide in the nearest bush or start running again. The first option presented me with stinging nettles and barbed wire, so I opted for the second one.

Run, walk, stop, run, walk, run, stop! It was a similar memory to that day at the Northampton Half the previous year. This was my pace for the next few miles until I reached the top of a hill. There was a drinks station strategically placed outside some pretty cottages and one of the only noisy spots on the quaint and quiet course. I stopped next to a lovely lady who offered me a cup of water and asked if I was OK. She assumed the hot weather had taken its toll on me while climbing the big hill in front of her. I took the cup from her, and she offered some jelly babies, which I also gratefully accepted. The moment of truth arrived. I wasn't sick. I felt sick, but the water and sugary, sticky sweets worked. She asked again if I was OK to continue, and then suddenly, I told her the news about Jules's cancer treatment. I have no idea why it came out of my mouth, but it did. She took my hand and gave me some words of encouragement and love. It was a blur, and I can't remember what she said or what she looked like, but it sent a wave of positivity through my body, and I suddenly felt energised. It may seem strange, but it was like the winter wonderland scene running through that forest in the Grizzly. Suddenly beauty shone through in a time of adversity. I took a few more jelly babies and downed my second cup of water before thanking her and turning to run off. I will never forget that moment. The remaining three miles of the route were downhill and then along a flat stretch of country road back to the finish at the village fair. I ran at a comfortable pace and crossed the line in just under two hours. The finish time was irrelevant today! I was mentally shattered!

The following day, Jules and some friends participated in a local Race for Life event, and I volunteered to help at the finish area. It was unbelievably emotional seeing so many ladies cross the line, and it was surreal knowing that pretty much everyone had been affected by cancer. They'd either been diagnosed or were wearing a tribute pinned to their top, naming someone who has. It hit home how many lives are affected by this disease. I felt incredibly proud of Jules and our friends as they crossed the line, dressed in pink. My stomach again was turning as I knew that Jules would probably struggle to walk a 10K when the treatment started in a few short weeks.

Tough Times
The weeks that followed involved more operations and a cancelled holiday. We love our travel and were given the go-ahead by the cancer nurse to book a holiday before Jules began her chemo the following month. However, she developed an infection the day after we booked it, and we were soon cancelling. We both needed a break, but it wasn't to be. It felt like the wind of change again. That old analogy of one step forward and two steps back would pop up from time to time. It was frustrating and soul destroying. We both sat in the conservatory and cried, hugging each other.

When I ran, I just tried to run as fast as I could. I think it was a combination of a release but also wanting to escape these challenges that life was giving. With all the travelling in my business coupled with this stress, I didn't realise it was taking its toll on me. I needed to be strong. Jules was strong, in fact, she was much stronger than me, but I kept putting on a brave face and dealing with it.

The treatment began, and it wasn't very pleasant. I'll never forget the first time we came home after the first round had been administered. We sat on the sofa, almost waiting for the sickness to kick in. Then it did, and it was heart-breaking. One minute, your wife is perfectly OK, and then next, she is feeling ill and being sick, and it's the worst sickness ever. Jules described it as being inside a washing machine while having a hangover. Add in a cocktail of drugs, including steroids, and suddenly my beautiful wife had been physically and mentally changed in a space of a few short months. Then there was the hair loss. Now, I will always unconditionally love Jules no matter what, but I understood how hard it was for her to lose her identity and the battering her confidence and self-esteem would take.

It was like sailing a small ship into the eye of a storm! Perhaps this is why I don't like running into a strong headwind. This storm would repeat on loop every three weeks as Jules returned for the next round of treatment. I'm not a fan of running on treadmills and this was like the worst treadmill ever.

I did my best to keep running and stay positive, and, in September, I did the second Northampton Half Marathon. Thankfully on the day, I had a much better run than the previous year and recorded a decent time. I remember the brilliant atmosphere on the course and then the love at the end of the race as my fellow club members were full of encouragement for everyone crossing the line. Jules was around halfway through the chemo side of the treatment, and everyone was so supportive. There was no escaping the question, 'How's Jules doing?' Those three words were the ones I heard the most and had to repeat the update to everyone who asked, which was draining. I could never reply and say I didn't want to talk about it. My friends were caring and I appreciated that.

Jules endured two hospital stays in the six rounds of chemotherapy, and they were bloody scary. The drugs administered were one of the harshest prescribed for any cancer treatment and can only be described as debilitating. It zaps the immune system, and your body has no fight to fend off infection. On the first trip to the hospital, Jules had a horrendous infection and her whole system began to shut down. Cue more intravenous drugs to add to the many drugs circulating around her body. The second stay involved a major blood transfusion. The analogy of sailing into a storm or running into a gale are ones I've overused in this chapter, but there is no other way to put it. To cap it off, I also suffered a collapsed lung in the autumn. While hosting an interval session at our club on a lovely sunny evening, I had to pull out of the session halfway through. By the time I'd walked home, I had the most horrendous pain in my lower back. The following day the doctor advised me to go to the hospital for a walk-in x-ray, and a week later, I was told I had a primary spontaneous pneumothorax. Yep, I had no idea what that meant either! A small tear in my lung caused air to escape and build up in my chest wall, causing the lung to collapse. It was just something else that we didn't need!

Thankfully, I didn't need a hospital stay, but it involved a giant needle stuck in my chest between my ribcage. Are you a squeamish person who doesn't like the sight of blood or the thought of big needles? If so, that's me too. I couldn't watch this episode, but thankfully the staff that did the treatment were brilliant and very understanding. Of course, I was apprehensive that this would impact my running. There's nothing worse than being injured and having to watch from the side-lines.

Kew the Storms

I remember the great storms of 1988. My mum and I spent the night at our static caravan in a local park called Overstone Solarium. I had some beautiful weekends there and met some great friends. We played football, went tracking through the woods, had barbecues and climbed trees. They were some idyllic, carefree summer days. The night the storm hit, the caravan rocked from side to side, and branches crashed down on the metal roof. The rain hammered against the windows, and the thunder and lightning were louder than when I saw AC/DC play Thunderstruck live. This thwarted an escape attempt to the car to drive home, so we had to stay put and hope for the best. After a sleepless night, the storm had subsided by morning, and I went exploring to survey the damage. Tree branches were scattered everywhere, and gardens had been destroyed. Fence panels littered grassy areas, probably hundreds of metres from their origin. Some caravans had been displaced from their foundations, and a few smaller ones had toppled over. Deep puddles remained as evidence of the torrential rain. I remember hearing about the damage this storm had ravaged in Kew Gardens. Thankfully, the trees that had fallen in Northamptonshire had missed our caravan that evening. Now I had a reason to be reminded of this storm.

Our life was about to begin again following the aftermath of the storm caused by the drugs and countless operations Jules had to endure. Her final round of chemo was scheduled before Christmas, and it was a relief but only the relief that the gale-force wind and torrential rain had stopped. It was now like the clean-up operation that followed. That day in 1988, park rangers drove around the caravan site removing offending branches from roads and people's properties. Some unfortunate people would've had to go through some lengthy insurance claims to pay for repairs to damaged property. Some trees would grow new branches, but some would face permanent damage. Our life would follow a similar pattern.

Thankfully, Jules could break this awful cycle of sickness that chemo brings, and, as the drug begins to leave the system, she could rebuild her strength. Once chemo stops, hair begins to grow again. I couldn't have imagined how a lady must feel, having beautiful long hair and then losing it in the blink of an eye. Now I understand it. Then there were the scars. Operations carry scars that take time to heal but will always be visible and sometimes painful forever, giving a constant reminder of the ordeal. Jules and I had both encountered life-changing traumas. Mine showed no physical scars, and the damage caused to my head was internal, only being picked up by a scan. Jules has visible scars, which can mostly be hidden by clothing and padding, but she sees them every day, and can act as a painful reminder of something that changes your life forever.

The most significant factor that remains forever is mental trauma. When a tree loses its branches in a storm, the branches probably won't grow again, but new shoots will appear on the tree. If the storm fells the whole tree, it will leave a hole in the ground and will never grow back and leave permanent damage. If I go back to Overstone today, I could probably pick out a hole in the ground where one of those trees stood over 30 years ago. Brain injury and breast cancer had left some big holes in our lives, and we now had to start looking at ways of rebuilding mentally. Ways to plant new trees and begin growing from scratch. I was under the common illusion of thinking that the end of chemo meant life could return as normal, but I knew it wouldn't be that simple. Jules had a low immune system, many scars and diminished confidence caused by multiple operations and medications. Lots of people see this defining moment as, that's it! It's over and life will return to normal. It couldn't be further from reality. We needed to start replanting those trees and nurturing the seeds to grow.

Running-wise, I finished my racing year with my 48th half marathon at the Bedford Harriers Half in a small village called Wootton on the edge of Bedford itself. I felt great on the day and was pleased with my time of just over 1:35. The goal was to reach 50 half marathons but doing 12 in the year was quite pleasing considering all the challenges we'd dealt with. Running sometimes gave me a great escape route, but it wasn't easy.

Work took me to the Isle of Wight for a week just before Christmas, and it was so difficult being away from home, even though I got to enjoy some festivities with some good people. At Christmas that year, I felt exhausted both mentally and physically. Jules felt the same, but her exhaustion was ten-fold to mine. We had a lovely day with the family on Christmas day, which was quite emotional. Part of you wants to celebrate the end of the treatment, but part of you knows that life will always be different.

———

Stories From the Field - Real Life Runners Bouncing Back

Sometimes it's difficult to bounce back from a big blow in life. A job loss, separation, illness or bereavement. We've all been there, haven't we? I caught up with some running friends who kindly opened up and shared personal stories.

Bex began with her emotional start to running, where she stared adversity in the face, *It was my most emotional race finish; I cried when I completed the Bedford 20 about five years ago. It was my first event a few months after having a full hysterectomy. I was told after the operation that you age quickly. You'll feel like you're 80. It's life-changing and the recovery will take over 18 months. My training was hard, and I didn't think I would be able to do this event. I turned up at the start trying to stay positive. About halfway around, my running friend, who wasn't taking part in the event, saw me and ran eight miles with me as she could see I was struggling. The mind can be a horrible negative place sometimes! She pushed me and made me realise that I can do anything if I put my mind to it. So, I cried as I crossed that line. Such a relief and achievement. The body is an amazing thing. And then I received hugs from other runners, people I didn't know. My cheerleader hubby is at every finish line now.'*

So many people have unique stories, but that is a whopper! Well done to Bex for sharing it and keep up the fantastic work and enjoy crossing many more finishing lines.

Another wonderful friend, Michelle, recently set up her own personal training business and has many stories to share. Michelle took up running and threw herself into the fun side of the sport. You'll regularly see her in fancy dress and hear her cheering everyone on at events. There's a good chance you'll also appear in a selfie on social media. She and her husband, Craig, run a fabulous podcast called *Running Tales*, which features fantastic interviews with runners from all over the world. I'd definitely recommend a listen. It was good to put the running shoe on the other foot (so to speak) and ask Michelle to share a snippet of her story.

'One of my best and most emotional finishes was after the Seville marathon, which was my first. I was just so happy straight after I completed it. However, it wasn't until I got home and walked through the front door that all this emotion came out. I burst into tears, and it hit me then what I had achieved for myself and the charity I was running for.'

Michelle continued and shared a similar experience to Rebecca. *'When I had my womb out, I vowed to myself to do another marathon, but before my first anniversary had passed, I was running the Paris Marathon, and it was boiling hot. I was determined to prove to myself mentally, more than anything, that I was strong and a survivor of a woman who can't have kids. When I crossed that line, the feeling was very much what I needed and made me stay positive to this day.'*

Michelle won't mind me saying that she makes me smile whenever I see her, as her personality is infectious. I've had loads of fun running with her at times. She arranges local themed runs including a shoe run around Northampton. Northampton has a famous shoemaking history, and the local council commissioned a project for local artists to paint large shoes that were strategically placed around the town. A group of us ran from one to another while sharing stories of the town's history. It was wonderful and great fun. I won't talk too much about how a security guard asked us to leave the shopping centre in town as we ran through it. Running in shopping centres isn't allowed.

Michelle is a resilient person who helps many others use running to help them overcome adversity. This includes coaching blind runners, individuals struggling with their weight and wheelchair athletes, to name a few.

I met Ben through supporting Northampton Town Football Club, and when I did my first Great North Run, he told me a tale of when he'd done it years before. He'd since stopped running as life sort of got in the way.

One day, I talked a few lads from the fans team into entering a local charity 10K at the beautiful Stowe House, a National Trust site on the edge of Northamptonshire and Buckinghamshire. Ben heard about the run and decided to join us, and we all made our way to the start line wearing our football shirts.

I'd been running for just over a year and was in training for my second Great North Run, so I was pretty excited about this event and introducing some friends to running events. Of course, Ben was a master and a pretty good runner from his past, and he announced that he'd return to running if he could break 45 minutes. Naturally, he did, and his love of the sport returned immediately.

At first, he joined my running club, Northampton Road Runners, but, back then, we weren't geared up to support runners who needed some structure in their training, so he left to join the town's top club, Rugby & Northampton and went on to win some local events. We enjoyed swapping running stories at events and, of course, at football matches too. Suddenly, his life took an unexpected turn, as he will share with you now;

'In 2014, I did three half marathons over three consecutive weekends. In the week leading up to the first one, I had a few health issues related to a medical condition I suffer from, which is nocturnal epilepsy. I had a few seizures in the week leading up to the first race, including the night before the event. It left me physically exhausted and in considerable pain just before I started them.

However, I did the races anyway and stupidly stuck to the plan of running all three under 90 minutes. As I finished the last one, I remember thinking, 'my body needs a break', as it felt different from usual at a cross-country race. I needed to sort and get epilepsy under control which I did, and took a break from running to do this. Once I was able to manage epilepsy through lifestyle and medication, I took a further break from running due to the invention of Netflix.

Thankfully I finally started running again in 2019 and rediscovered track running in 2021. The specific training for this is ideal for me in ensuring a build-up of physical exhaustion doesn't occur, which for me is a major trigger for seizures.

I did miss running a little, particularly the local road race series, but I knew figuring out how to control my epilepsy was more important. Starting track running gave me a new drive and passion for the sport again, more so as track racing was what I did as a child.

Half Man, Half Marathon

I told some of my fellow club runners the same thing I said to Mark years ago, 'If I go under 2:25 minutes for 800 metres, I'll take up track racing'. I did, of course, and the rest, as they say, is history.'

Having chatted with Ben and gone through his story, some real key moments hit home for me. I pushed myself to hit some good times and PBs during 2015, which I'll share with you in the next chapter. I guess sometimes we need to slow life down or adapt to suit what our bodies can handle.

Thoughts Running Through the Mind

In this chapter, I guess running summed up life in general. Just like in that cross country, running can take you through cow poo. Metaphorically, life is sometimes going to throw some poo at you, but you must just dig in and push on. There was also a phrase that mentioned peeing in the wind, yep, I know, another bodily fluid analogy. Running into the wind is like sailing into it, but the sail's set will determine the sailboat's direction. Sometimes we must sail on (or, in my case, run on) when the storm is raging.

As Bex, Michelle and Ben shared, they had to show their resilience while making some significant adjustments to their lives. Sometimes, it isn't always about what happens to you but it's how you respond to a situation that will determine your success.

Think about moments in your life where you've had to bounce back and be stronger and more determined. Perhaps that time is now? Maybe you're facing adversity and it feels like the wind is in your face and the life poo is deep. What's your first step? In the case of running, it could be slowing down and walking for a bit. Maybe you could slow down and take stock of the situation. Perhaps a waterproof running coat or a pair of gloves would help. What armour of protection would aid you in this situation?

Perhaps it's a situation that isn't running-related! Maybe reaching out to a friend or family member or attending a peer support group. Maybe even offering forgiveness to someone who may have wronged you. Of course, every situation is complex, and there isn't a one size fits all answer.

It's OK not to be OK

Mental health has been a hot topic for many years, but it's becoming more widely accepted in the UK to open up and talk about it. However, a typically British demeanour is to shrug it off and deal with it.

Could you open up and talk to a family member or a friend? Maybe there's something that irritates you about them, and you could both work on a solution together. Perhaps it's the other way around, and you could be open to some changes and compromises to create harmony in relationships.

Don't forget that this works the other way around too. You may have a habit or trait that irritates someone else, perhaps your partner or family. We sometimes hide behind the phrase, '*Oh, that's just the way I am, I can't change*'. This, in truth, is rubbish, we can change habits if we really want to. So, think about your irritation and how you could change it for those around you. Honestly, you'll feel a much better person for it.

This is quite a deep and personal final thought in this chapter.

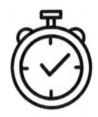

8. Personal Bests

Do you know someone who is fascinated by sequences? You know, that person who gets excited when the date was the 12th of December in 2012 and managed to capture a photo of their clock displaying the time of 12:12? The sequence would show 12:12 12/12/12!

Admit it; perhaps you're one of those who loves pointless stuff like that. OK, I'm going to confess here, I'm that guy too! My favourite time of day is 12:34 pm because I love the sequence. It has absolutely nothing to do with the time of day, but I get a little moment of satisfaction from seeing that number. It's the same when the car milometer clocks over the next 10,000 miles or when I ran a parkrun of precisely 20 minutes. I was a little gutted the latter wasn't a second quicker though.

If you're a runner, you'll also resonate with the obsession to round up your running distance to an exact mileage. Yep, at our running club, many members loop around the car park trying to get their watches to an exact five-mile reading for example.

My nan used to have a saying, 'Little things please little minds!' so I guess that always referred to my love of straightforward stuff like this.

My goal for 2015 was to run 15 half marathons. I called it 15 in 15! Simple really; what else would I call it? There was no reason for doing this other than a personal challenge. We run a part-time network marketing business, and I started the year speaking at a prominent local seminar where Jules and I were asked to share our story. Unfortunately, Jules was poorly on the day, so I spoke on my own. I mentioned my running and personal goal to do the 15 in 15, so I guess I was committed to over a thousand people.

Desperate to help Jules regain her confidence and get our lives on track, I went into overdrive. We had a trip down to London to celebrate Jules's birthday, but I decided to take it further and book some flights to Thailand. We needed a break, and this seemed an ideal place to go, away from crowds and people we knew. Jules was apprehensive and quite nervous about it, but I assured her everything would be fine. Her hair had begun to grow back, and the scars were healing, but this treatment is cruel and batters your self-esteem. I knew how difficult it would be, but despite everything, we had a wonderful few weeks on a mini tour of the island of Phuket.

A couple of days after flying back from Bangkok via Bahrain, I was standing on the start line of the Berkhamsted Half Marathon in slightly cooler temperatures. Well, when I say slightly cooler, I meant a hell of a lot cooler.

It was a crazy few days! We left Bangkok on a late flight and landed at London Heathrow at 6:00am on a Saturday because of the time difference. As the plane began its descent, I began to ponder the possibility of making the parkrun back in Northampton. We had to factor in a ninety-minute drive after leaving the plane, clearing passport control, picking up our bag and boarding the bus to the car park. The plane had to loop the airport twice before being cleared to land, which made things a bit tighter. Passport control was surprisingly quiet, and we breezed through. As soon as we got in the car, I started to change into my running kit, and Jules drove the M25 and then the M1 northbound. The satnav said the ETA was 9:08am. No drama, that added to the challenge! Our nephew and niece, Neil and Lois, had been running the parkrun regularly back then, and they were planning to be there that day. My goal was now to catch them both. Messages flew back and forth as we continued our journey on the quiet motorways.

Don't ask me how but we pulled into the street next to the start of the parkrun at 8:51am, and I casually wandered to the start with minutes to spare. It was a combination of a minor traffic delay clearing and Jules not breaking the speed limit (honestly).

The following day, I was in Hertfordshire for the Berkhamsted Half. Berko, listen to me sounding like a local, has fond memories for me. Not only is it a beautiful course, but it was also the location of what was my current PB at the time. I ran 1:33:37 and did the last mile in under six minutes. I was on fire that day, and the super-fast downhill finish helped me to a time I was immensely proud of.

One of the most amazing things about running is the feeling of a personal best time. When you run your first-ever event, you suddenly have a benchmark and something to beat, should you so wish. It's exciting doing a new distance because you're guaranteed a PB. I also find that many newer runners quickly get the buzz as their times fall alongside their increased confidence in running and fitness. In my first year of running, I racked up six PBs in six consecutive races of different distances. I then did a couple of challenging events where it would've been difficult to sustain that run. There are also a few dangers of the PB though. One is the plateau effect, the period when your times can start to level out or even slow down. Sometimes people give up or lose their passion for running. A plateau in any pastime can lead to a person losing interest, of course, so it's good to keep setting and evaluating new goals. Another danger is injury. I've seen friends sustain long-term injuries by constantly pushing too hard and too quickly.

Thankfully, I've never suffered any serious running-related injury. I think my freak head injury made up for that in a big way. I have been hugely disappointed with some of my times in the past, especially not breaking four hours in a marathon. However, when I look back, I am immensely proud to have run London four times and Paris too. They are incredible memories, and the finish times seem irrelevant now.

In 2015, I wondered if I could record a PB in the 15 half marathons that lay in wait. I hadn't planned every event because I know things come up in life, but I had a rough idea of some that I wanted to do. Some of the excitement in my goals is not being too clinical and structured; it's more exciting to me, not having the whole journey planned out, leaving room for exciting last-minute changes or spontaneous decisions.

Berko was great! I loved it. It was my first half of the year. At ten miles, the route goes through the Ashridge Estate, a stately home sitting at the top of some amazing countryside. Once you leave the estate, the road winds through stunning woodland before that fast, final mile. In the forest, deer run free along the quiet country lanes, not caring that runners were rushing past. It was a truly magical moment in the late winter sunshine. A combination of two weeks in Thailand and 15 hours on a plane didn't make ideal preparations for a PB. My legs were heavy, and I was over five minutes from the target time. I confess I wasn't expecting a PB that day though. It may have had something to do with the epic journey back from south-east Asia and jet lag that put the kybosh on that.

Failing to Plan is Planning to Fail

Talking of preparation, my next half fell afoul of a lack of it. I have friends who lay their kit out the night before and even have their race number readily pinned to their vest. I sometimes throw all my stuff in a bag in the morning and pretty much get it right. Half marathon number 50 wasn't that time. Have you ever read some instructions loosely and then realised perhaps you should've paid a little more attention?

I arrived at the village of Naseby to run the Battlefield Half. The event was named after the Battle of Naseby that took place in Northamptonshire in June 1645. During the first English Civil War, Oliver Cromwell defeated the Royalist army under Charles I. Now I'm going to stop with the history stuff there, as civil wars and that subject were never my strong point. However, I now know that the run of 16.45 miles from Naseby is to commemorate the battle.

Anyway, I'm not avoiding my point on purpose here. For some reason, I thought the Battlefield Half would be run around the battlefields, and field was the keyword that led me to believe it was off-road. I turned up in my old, battered trail shoes only to find it was run entirely on country roads. 13.1 miles later, my feet were swearing at my lack of instruction, care, and attention. It was a painful way to celebrate my 50th half marathon, but thankfully there was no damage done, and I ran two actual off-road events, in the same trail shoes, in the following few weeks.

I was getting closer to that elusive PB, and my fifth half of the year was one of my other favourites (I have many, I know), the Bournemouth Bay Half again. I've been blessed with lovely weather when running there and this event was no different. I crossed the line just over a minute short of my target time.

If there are many favourite places I want to run, Milton Keynes isn't one of them. A few weeks after the seaside, I was running around MK for the half distance of the marathon festival. Close to home and a flat course with cheering spectators and open green spaces, what's not to love? I've always found Milton Keynes is one of the very few places where I can easily get lost, and I don't know why. The main roads are all too similar, with too many roundabouts and few unique landmarks. Inside the grid system, every route seems almost too flat, which means I feel the need to run fast. At the risk of upsetting anyone from Milton Keynes, I'll tell you what I love about it. Aside from a potential PB, it's a popular running venue that's always well attended. It's a vibrant and ambitious place, now an official city and the local authority seems open-minded to support any new and exciting venture. Sadly, one of those includes their football team. As a Northampton fan, they're our closest rivals. Anyway, back to the positives, Milton Keynes also shares my initials, and I was excited for the MK Half. It was a chance to push for my goal. Besides the crowds, there aren't too many distractions along the route, and the roads are wide enough to get a good pace.

From the start, I was flying and soon focused on my target of a PB. As each mile passes, I usually do calculations in my head to see what time I think I'll cross the line. Breaking 1:33 seemed a possibility as I passed each mile marker. Occasionally I heard a local friend call my name out, but there was no time for stopping today. The last couple of miles are a bit of a killer. The finish line is inside the football ground, but you have to pass the stadium, do a lap around a lake, and then head back inside to complete a lap of the pitch. I had to forget that act of cruelty and dig in. Passing 12 miles, I worked out I had around nine minutes to get to the finish. The May sunshine was starting to beat down as my legs began to feel like jelly, but I dug in, raced into the arena, lapped the pitch, and crossed the line. Ten steps later, I sprawled out on the carpet-like grass at the side of the pitch and paused before the moment of truth. My watch read 1:32:33. I'd done it! A steward then ran over to tell me to get off the pitch. To be honest, I didn't care; I was in dreamland and it was my moment!

My journey out of Stadium:MK was much happier than the previous year. There was no stopping in the corridor to mentally rest and stare at the wall. This time, it was more of a slow walk with a big smile on my face.

Back to Reality

Although things were going well on the running circuit, my life felt the opposite. Seemingly insignificant things were stressful, and I became agitated very easily. Driving was tiring and, I mean, more tiring than ever. My love of visiting schools around the country was becoming more and more difficult. Being a motivational speaker, you must be on your game from the minute you walk through the venue gates to the minute you leave. My game face was on, but my mind wasn't there. It was confusing. Jules had finished her treatment, and we could do some of the wonderful things we wanted to do in life again. It didn't make sense, so I just pushed on. Work started to quieten down in June, so I just put it down to being busy and dismissed it, thinking everything would be fine.

Over the summer, I did more races and got some great times. In an off-road 10K, I was just over ten seconds away from a PB, which was amazing given the challenging, undulating course. I also recorded my fastest parkrun of 19:28 and ran a 5:50 mile, one second off a PB at that distance.

The summer holidays were over, but before I began my road trips to schools around the country, it was time for the Northampton Half Marathon again. As I made my way to the start line in the town centre, which was a short walk from home, I felt slightly nervous about the disaster from two years previously. The butterflies soon flew away from my tummy as I arrived at The Guildhall, Northampton's beautiful town hall building and dropped my bag off. I felt focused and full of belief, all the uncertainty in my life seemed to disappear at that moment. Ten, nine, eight, seven, six… the countdown began, and I hovered my finger over the watch button, ready for the off. Five, four, three… I glanced up and looked at the quick runners right before me. Two, one… gooooooooooooooooo! We were off!

I flew through the first few miles as the route left the town centre and headed towards a large park, known as The Racecourse. In the late 1800s, it was a horse racing track, but meetings ceased in 1904 as the course was deemed unsafe due to a fatal accident involving some spectators. The park is now the largest open space in the town and home of the Northampton parkrun. I've felt privileged to have this on my doorstep, and it's wonderful that the half marathon route had been changed to run within a few hundred metres from my home. Naturally, Jules stood there, cheering me on, next to my mum, who lives in the same street as us. It's so wonderful seeing your family cheering, and it gives you that extra boost which I'm sure many of my running friends will relate to. That boost continued as I powered around the course. One of the things I love about doing a local event is seeing friends and hearing familiar voices. People shouting out words of encouragement.

After another loop through the town centre, the route heads out into the countryside via a large industrial estate and then up a hill known as Brackmills Hill. This is named after the industrial estate but does get called other names that may be unprintable. For the first time in the course, runners are hit by a sharp climb which is quite energy-sapping. Today though, I felt like I was gliding up it and checked my pace on my watch. It hadn't decreased despite the climb.

The cursed ten-mile marker had been moved slightly to incorporate the new route, which meant I didn't have to pass puke point, as I referred to it. As I made my way towards the next mile marker, I started to get goosebumps knowing I was on for a PB. The mental statistical maths calculations had been going through my mind for some time now, and I knew I could make it. The last few miles are tricky though. After ten miles on roads, the route suddenly veers onto an old disused railway line which is a little rough underfoot. If that isn't challenging enough, the last three-quarters of a mile is through a stunning park known as Delapré. This is the site of another memory of my childhood. My nan, the one who would take me to Bournemouth, would bring me to Delapré, and I'd run around the gardens, which were surrounded by tall trees. It was a little like a secret garden where a child with a vivid imagination like mine could get lost in fun and magical thoughts. I was now an adult, running through these same trees and hearing the noise from the PA system at the finish line. Underfoot, the ground was loose dirt paths, but I was now invincible as I emerged from the woodland and made the final loop of the lawn in front of the beautiful Delapré Abbey. Northampton is blessed with many open spaces, and it's humbling to think this place is only a mile from the town centre. My arms were raised, and I tapped the Northampton Road Runners badge on my chest, mimicking a footballer showing his dedication to his club. I then took two steps, accepted my medal and dropped to my knees in delight. I'd heard Jules cheering as I approached the line, so I knew I had to go and find her immediately. I looked at my watch and it read 1:31:47! Yesssss! I cheered loud enough for me to hear but not loud enough to cause a spectacle of myself. I jumped to my feet and realised that I probably didn't have as much energy as I'd had earlier that morning, so I stepped forward gingerly and found Jules. I was so proud to have a PB at my hometown half marathon now, and I'd exorcised the ghosts of 2013. Puke hill, you can go and do one!

I was on top of the world as we walked back into town and made our way to Nando's for some food. Sometimes, eating after a run takes me a while, but today I was so hungry. After a spicy bean wrap, some fries, nuts and a celebratory beer later, we made our way home.

Back to the Start

A week later, it was time to go back to where it all began, the Great North Run. Our niece Lois had entered the event, and I'd decided to make it a family trip up north to support her by running it too. OK, there was a bit of the old fear of missing out, or FOMO syndrome too. My stepson Russell and daughter-in-law Roxanne also lived in Darlington, so we didn't have to stay in Banana Joe's in Whitley Bay like that first GNR experience. Roxanne was heavily pregnant with their firstborn Isaac, so I headed off to Newcastle with Lois and her husband Oli on the morning of the run.

Lois was nervous, and I felt like a pro, so I took the lead after Oli dropped us in the city centre or Toon as the locals call it. It was a buzz to walk through the crowds of runners and see a helicopter flying overhead. After a long wait in the toilet queues, we wished each other good luck and headed to our respective starting pens. As mentioned earlier, these big events have sections for runners based on their predicted finish time, and this time, I'd managed to get into Pen B, the first one behind the elites. With minutes to go to the start time, I pushed my way right to the front of that pen, probably uncharacteristically offending a few people on the way who probably thought I was being rude. No sooner had I caught sight of the elite runners than the race countdown was complete, and we were on our way. Fresh from my PB a week before, I was daring to dream today. It was wonderful to get ahead of the mass crowds and make the most of the sparsely populated roads. At my previous two Great North Run events, it was impossible to put your arm out in any direction and not encounter a fellow runner. Today was different; there was space to settle into a good pace.

The crowd were as raucous as ever as I left Newcastle, crossed the Tyne Bridge and made my way through Gateshead. I passed the familiar sign that reads, 'You've Reached Halfway, Have a Great Second Half of the Race'. My watch read 44 minutes and 50 seconds! I looked again in disbelief as it was now ticking over 45 minutes. At this pace, I would break the ninety-minute barrier. More cheering crowds, more offers of jelly babies and more sounds of the Blaydon Races and other musical classics from the bands on the route. The inevitable soon happened though. It's a big ask to run two stupidly quick races in two weeks, and, suddenly, my previous week's glory decided to remind my legs that this was probably not going to happen. At mile 10, I decided to slow down and look for the beer guys. Why ever not? I couldn't maintain this pace, and it was starting to drop. Spoiler alert, I didn't get a PB that day, but the thing I was most gutted about was that I missed the beer stop. The two chaps handing out little cups of beer came into my sight just as I'd passed them. Tempted to turn around but realistic that this would really annoy runners around me, I carried on.

The last mile along the coast road in South Shields seemed like four miles. The finish line just wouldn't get any closer, and I was now ready to finish the Great North Run. It's been nice knowing you, but I want to go home! The left leg was saying to the right, come on, can't we just have a bloody rest right now? 800 metres to go! Seriously, that's half a mile; I just want to sit down. Sod off you cheering crowds, you've no idea how much this is hurting now. Pushing through the pain barrier past the 400 metres sign. What! That's a quarter of a mile, that's still too far. Yeah, I'll give you a high five mate, do you know how much energy that takes when my legs feel like this. Ooh, look, some kids wanting a high five. Nah, too much effort. 200 metres to go. Hmm, the line is getting closer now; I can almost touch it. Push, push, push... shall I sprint to the line? Erm, no, there's no point, the PB has gone, and it's not worth messing myself up. Ooh, there's the finish, yessssss, we've done it! Thank you, legs, you held up. Thank you for my medal, friendly, smiley volunteer, yes, please, I'd love a seat. OK, I know I can't sit here, I'll keep moving. Ha, that'll do, I'm going to sit down here! Yes, finally, a rest spot. The voices and emotions in my head did the talking, and I couldn't be disappointed to be three minutes slower than last week in Northampton. I finished in 1,380th place, the top three per cent of over 40,000 runners.

It was time for a few weeks off before another trip to Bournemouth for more lovely memories on the south coast. The rest did me good as I was agonisingly close to another PB, a mere seven seconds slower than Northampton. On the day as the early October morning shone onto the sea, which was so calm that it resembled a pond. My dad, little brother and step mum, who also ran the half, met us in the Central Gardens after the event, and we sat in the sunshine just wearing t-shirts. Jules and I said our goodbyes after a nice meal, but it was so lovely that we drove a couple of hundred metres down the road before stopping and checking into a hotel for an extra night on the south coast. This is another wonderful thing about running, it can take you to some lovely places to add to the experience. It was also half marathon number twelve of the year making 60 in total.

I had three half marathons left to run. St Neots and Lanzarote had been entered for November and December. I wanted to do a special final race, so Lanza seemed ideal. The missing link was number 13. The reason is both

Jules's sons were expecting to become dads imminently, so it was difficult to commit to entering an event in late October and early November. The one I'd earmarked was the Lode Half, the lovely small event I ran in the gale-force wind the year before. Our granddaughter, Thea, was born at the end of October, so Lode was on. It would be OK because I could enter on the day, just like last year. Arriving at the race HQ, I was told the race was full. Oh poo, were my words (or something to that effect). After a bit of explaining, smiling, pleading and begging, the organisers found a solution. They first suggested I do the five-mile fun run, but I'd explained my 15 in 2015 goal, and they thought I was mad enough to bend over backwards. I'd also said I was dedicating it to my granddaughter and calling it the 'Thea Run'! They knew of a local runner who'd pulled out, so they gave me their number and changed the details on the timing chip.

Lining up at the start, I made my way to a small group of runners and placed myself in the second row. I was keen to get off to a good start but didn't want to run off into the lead as I was sure there would be some quicker runners in the race. After the countdown, we were off and took in a lap of the field, running on grass, before heading out through the sleepy village of Lode. Passing a couple of locals out walking their dogs or going for the Sunday paper, I soon settled into a comfortable pace.

The route turned off of a country road onto a narrow track and then along some narrow farm tracks and trails. There was an air of mystery with the soon to be winter fog hanging just above the ground. Cows grazed, blissfully unaware of the runners flying past. And I was flying. Each glance of the watch showed my pace was below seven-minute miles. I was excited but kept calm, knowing I wasn't yet at the halfway point.

The only part of the course that wasn't flat was a humpback bridge over a river and that did nothing to take away my pace. After navigating that, it was more flat country roads before the turning point at halfway. Thankfully, there was no wind this year, it was calm and still. I was pleased as I put my head down and began retracing my steps back towards Lode.

With a mile to go, the course re-joined the main country road back into the village. Another look at the watch and I knew the PB was on. I had way over ten minutes to complete the last mile and started to get excited about breaking the 1:30 barrier. However, my legs were really starting to feel the pace and I felt like I was slowing slightly. It was time to dig in. The runner in front began to pull away but I didn't care, I had no desire to catch him. This was my own race.

A left turn, along a gravel track that led to some householder's driveways, a quick shimmy through a narrow pathway and I was back on the field. The lap of the field seemed more like a mile than a few hundred yards. Attempting a sprint finish in the final few steps, I was exhausted.

After finishing the race, I went and found the organiser and asked her if I could give her a big hug of thanks. She obliged and asked me how I'd got on. I was delighted that the 'Thea Run' was a personal best. The conditions were ideal that day. No wind combined with a flat course gave me a finish time of 1:30:12, and it remains my PB to this day. People often ask if I'm gutted that I couldn't have knocked off an extra second per mile, but my answer is always no. I'm immensely proud of that time.

Our grandson Isaac was born a couple of weeks later, so I dedicated the St. Neots Half to him and called it the Isaac Run. There would be no personal best that day. It was a strong headwind from seven miles in, and I've told you my thoughts of running into the wind. The 'Isaac Run' did become even more special in years to come, and you'll find out why later in the book.

I achieved my goal while on holiday in Lanzarote in December 2015 and felt all kinds of emotions. Joyous at achieving my goal of the fifteen half marathons and, although I was tired physically and shattered mentally but satisfied from a year of personal bests. It had been a fantastic year because we'd crammed so much stuff in. Not only the running, but we'd been to Thailand, Corfu, Berlin, where we saw AC/DC, Italy and Lanzarote. There had been so many highs. Jules had some of her confidence and energy back, and her hair was growing back following her treatment. However, I just couldn't shake this foggy feeling around me. Life was good, and when I experienced those high moments, they were high. Unfortunately, there were a lot of low points too. I'd been back to the neurological department at Northampton General Hospital and been told that this could be down to anxiety and depression. Anxiety, I got it. That's why I'd experience panic attacks, but depression, you're having a laugh; people with depression don't run PBs and have loads of holidays, they avoid social situations, and their lives are inconsistent. Oh, hang on a minute…

The Anxious Runner

These things were happening to me. One minute I was on top of the world, running a personal best in a race or visiting a beauty spot on holiday with my lovely wife. The next, I'm a quivering wreck and hiding away. I'd be rocking to the band AC/DC but then not wanting to be in a noisy room with a handful of family members. I loved being a motivational speaker, but when I was arriving at gigs, I couldn't wait to be back home. If I had to stay away overnight, I felt helpless and needy, like a child separated from a parent for the first time in their life.

Fatigue was horrendous! Bizarrely, I couldn't sleep some nights, and couldn't wake up on others. Brain injury fatigue and being tired from lack of sleep is very different, but I diddn't understand them. Car journeys would sometimes take ages because I'd have to keep pulling over to service stations and sleep. Driving at night was harder to concentrate on long journeys. My memory was affected, and I struggled to remember really important bits of information but could remember useless facts. Friends would also say how much weight I'd lost, but I dismissed it as rubbish. I just wanted to get on with life, and when Jules asked if I was OK or suggested a solution, I'd just snap back and say I was fine. This was also strange because I'm not a naturally snappy or stressy person. I just wanted the old me back all of the time. I've been one for being my personal best, but not just on the running circuit.

Family members and close friends kept asking Jules what was wrong with me. They said I was vacant or withdrawn. Inside, I felt nervous in situations I usually thrived in, except while running races.

After another visit to the neurology department, I'd been given a referral to Headway, the charity that supports people with brain injury. I'd heard of them when friends raised money for them while running events like the London Marathon. They are a wonderful organisation, but I didn't feel like it fitted at first. While visiting monthly drop-in centres, there were people in wheelchairs and using walking sticks. A pang of guilt washed over me because I was the fit, active guy who runs half marathons and drives all over the country. This was a big case of imposter syndrome as I wasn't yet familiar with the term 'hidden disability'.

Once I completed my 15th half of the year, I didn't race again for another six months, other than parkruns. We made another trip to Thailand, and upon our return, my lung collapsed again. This made me nervous about pushing myself and added another thing to knock my confidence and raise anxiety. The first time around, I could deal with it, but it happened again and made me feel vulnerable. I knew Jules and my family and friends were also concerned that I could end up in hospital or have some long-term damage, but they encouraged me to get out of the door again. I guess the fear was relatively short-lived though as I'm always determined to do things I love.

Stories From the Field - Real Life Runners and Their PBs

The personal best is a real key, not only in running but in life too. We live in a world where it's difficult to avoid self-comparison and find others who appear much better than us. Focusing on being your best is key, so I spoke to some runners and asked them what their best ever running performance was and how they felt when they achieved it.

Times and PBs can be really important to us runners; they're a good benchmark for measuring how we are improving. Becci said her finest moment was, '*Achieving my goal of a sub-four-hour marathon at Manchester was the best feeling ever. I had trained so hard, and everything went right on the day. I didn't feel emotional when I finished. I felt a great sense of achievement and was so proud of myself.*'

I instantly told Becci I was jealous as the sub-four-hour marathon has always eluded me. That could be interpreted as a bit of self-comparison there, couldn't it?

Joanne talked about her marathon and even though she didn't reach her time goal, it was still big personal best. '*I ran a marathon in 4:31, which was so close to my goal. I wanted to break 4:30 but my training didn't go quite to plan, so I was more than happy to be so close. The time has become less important to me though, as I was immensely proud of completing the distance. I entered again, and at that minute, a time goal didn't really bother me. However, we'll see what happens when it gets closer. We can all be competitive with ourselves!*'

Nicola was also buzzing more about the event experience than the time, '*Definitely completing my first marathon in Manchester last year. The feeling when I crossed the line was amazing. I loved every minute! I've never felt anything like it; I was on a high for days!*'

Running isn't just about marathons, of course, but staying on the 26.2 theme, I recently spoke to a friend, Sue. She shared, '*Running the London Marathon in 2003 was special. I had never entered any running event before but received a letter from the Marie Curie charity just before Christmas to say I had a place to run the London Marathon the following April. I'd actually forgotten I had applied. The charity had previously given end-of-life care to my mum. So, I bought my first-ever running shoes and began training. At the time, I lived on a farm and running around the area was beautiful.*

I completed my first ever running event, and I am proud to say I ran all the way and never stopped. Also, I didn't lose a toenail or get any blisters, an achievement in itself. It was the year Paula Radcliffe set her world record. I remember being on such an emotional high for weeks after.'

As you know, a half marathon is my favourite distance. Here are a few stories from runners who had an emotional finish to their first events at the 13.1 mile distance. Kathy said, '*Completing my first half marathon after post-life-changing surgery. It took three years of recuperating, so it was a wonderful experience for me.*'

Chrissy also shared a wonderful way to finish her race, '*Running my second half marathon at Milton Keynes; I ran into the stadium and the arms of my eldest grandson at the end. It was the best reward possible.*'

Mark went a lot further in distance for his favourite running moment. It also hit a lot of special emotions for him. *'My biggest running achievement was planning my training and completing Rat Race The Wall, a 70 Mile Ultra. This was despite having a meniscus tear and being told not to run it! The feeling of finishing with a fellow club runner was amazing! I felt so emotional, happy but wrecked all in one, which made me cry and think of my dad. It was on his birthday too.'*

Andy achieved international honours shortly after he retired. What an achievement and one showing that age is no barrier. *'I was honoured to represent England at the Tenby 10K. It was definitely the best running moment for me. My England running shirt is going in a frame and will be proudly hanging on the wall.'*

Neil took part in a 24-hour relay event recently and described his favourite running moment, *'The last lap of Endure recently with a group of lovely people was indescribable. We'd had no sleep Saturday night, but the gods were with me Sunday morning, and I felt that I was flying. It was probably the quickest and last of my four laps and the best run I will have all year!'*

We heard Ben's story in the chapter Running in the Wind. He added an extra line I saved for this chapter because it made me smile. *'I once came first in a parkrun. I looked at my watch and thought it was way off a PB, but the person in second wasn't catching me, so I decided to milk it and did a cartwheel over the finish line.'* What an exhibitionist, hey?

As mentioned, running isn't just about times but nor is it necessarily about races. James summed this up in his year-long challenge. *'I managed to run the equivalent of Lands' End to John O' Groats last year after originally setting the goal of running 1,000km. I got into the flow after just missing my target the previous year. I got injured at the start of this year, and it's amazing how your goals change; I ended up completing over 1,407km.'*

One runner, I won't use their name, gave probably the simplest example. *'This may seem silly but coming back to running after struggling with my mental health for a period. The first step felt like the hardest, but now enjoying running again.'* It's not silly. Getting out and running is sometimes just what is needed.

———

Thoughts Running Through the Mind

In a world of social media, we see the so-called perfect pictures of life by scrolling through celebrities' feeds. Fashion magazines have long since painted an image of the size six body or six-pack abs. Then television has also given us reality TV that is probably far from being real. It's hard to escape these influences. Even running magazines can contain pictures of super-fit and slim runners effortlessly making their way around a course without a bead of sweat on their bodies.

Having worked in the education system for several years, I've seen teens and young adults measured on grades and statistical results, which significantly have a significant impact on their adult lives.

Think about how to focus on being your best in life. How could you avoid putting down your excellent achievements because of self-comparison? Is there a way to find someone better than you at something and use them as an inspiration? How could they help you to achieve your goal?

One thing I've learned through running a business is that I've been happy to be a small enterprise. Employing hundreds of members of staff and working long hours for the reward of lots more money isn't something on my radar. Self-comparison and imposter syndrome have kicked in many times, especially when I've felt I should be doing more.

In my running, I've also drooled at friends' running times, wishing I could run a half marathon five or ten minutes quicker or discipline myself to push harder and further.

So, how do you rein yourself in and aim for your absolute best? In the Thoughts Running Through the Mind sections throughout this book, you will have noticed a theme around writing down goals and thoughts. This part is no different, think about your goal and what it is that you want to achieve and then write down who your inspiration is to achieve it.

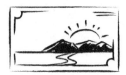

9. Running to the Beach

The last chapter was a little deep about mental health and life's adversities, so let's take you on holiday. Do you ever have that idyllic moment in your mind? You know, perhaps the one where you're watching a sunset, sitting on a beach while sipping a cocktail? As well as running, I love to travel, as you can guess from the stories so far. In fact, as far as addictions go, both are very high up on my scale, along with chocolate. So, I guess an idyllic moment for me is running along the beach while watching the sunset and then sipping a cocktail when I've finished.

Jules and I have had many trips, from weekend city breaks to long backpacking trips. Experiencing different cultures, climates, scenery and cuisine is absolutely divine. So, what could be better than adding running into the travel pot?

As mentioned, to finish the 15 in 2015, I wanted the final run to be special, so I opted for a week in the Canary Islands and to race at the end of the week. Lanzarote it was, for some winter sunshine.

Another couple of things I learnt was a week of holiday food and beer affects your running performance. Yeah, obviously! Also, cycling 30 odd miles on a basic, clapped-out hired bike is sapping on the legs. Well, what did I expect? Also, Lanzarote can be hot in the morning, even in December. One more, Spanish to English translations can be mismatched at times. So, when I boarded the bus to take me to the start at 8:00am, two hours before the race began, I didn't realise that it was the first bus laid on by the organisers and not the only bus. Loads of us Brits were standing there, chatting away for a couple of hours in the early morning sun, all realising we'd made the same error.

It was wonderful though. I met a lovely lady from Scotland at the start. We chatted like a pair who'd been friends forever before the run and we still keep in touch on Facebook now.

The run itself was fabulous. It hugged the coast from start to finish and provided a welcome distraction from the hot sun as the race wore on. There was a marathon distance that passed by the start of the half, at their halfway point, before we began. Half marathon runners then repeated the same experience, running through the 10K start line in the island's capital, Arrecife and meeting the 5K start line as the route approached the resort town of Costa Teguise on the island. These memories stuck in my mind and gave me such a buzz as I tucked into a huge post-run pizza in the afternoon sun. Finding a bar for an evening pint, fellow tourists praised my so-called mad achievement of running while on holiday.

Romance on the Run

My first experience of crossing the sea and racing in another country was a long weekend visit to Paris for the Paris Marathon, as mentioned earlier. A few days before the event, we boarded Eurostar at Waterloo, and the excitement levels were high. I'd been through the Channel Tunnel once but only on a coach, so I only got to experience the very dark part of the journey. Jules hadn't been on Eurostar before, though. Travelling by train is magical; looking out of the window and seeing the world as you fly past at great speed. We'd been to Paris before but, having loved it then, it was an absolute delight to return.

After a day of exploring, a handful of running buddies from the running club arrived the following morning and we met up in Montmartre for a spot of lunch. Bizarrely, the food in the restaurant was awful given that France is known for its fabulous cuisine. Thankfully, it was a one-off on this trip as we found some much nicer places.

The marathon itself was a unique experience. At the start, I was lined up in the 4:00-4:15hr pen, ready to go. It took ages to get going as the runners were set off in waves about ten minutes apart. By the time I crossed the start line, I'd been waiting for almost an hour but soon settled into a reasonable pace along the Champs Elysée. Suddenly, a photographer jumped out in front of me and started snapping away with his camera, and I had to pretty much run around him.

The Parisian public came out in their droves to cheer runners on, but some didn't quite seem in the spirit. I remember reaching ten miles and hearing the sound of a motorised scooter getting louder. The crowd of runners were shocked to see the motorist riding his moped straight through the middle of the course into oncoming athletes.

Around halfway, in the Bercy district, an elderly gentleman crossed the road with his shopping bag in his hand, and runners swerved around him. He angrily gestured towards the crossing lights, pointing out they showed the green man, and he had every right to cross. I wasn't sure how he expected tens of thousands of runners to get out of his way on this one day of the year. It was very amusing, to say the least.

Aside from the event running out of water in the final seven miles, Paris was a wonderful experience. Having run past so many world-famous landmarks, I had the bug to visit some more countries and combine my love of running with my love of travel. Jules was also sold on the travel element.

The day after the marathon, we decided to have a trip up the Eiffel Tower and meet up with our running club friends. At the top of the tower, we pulled out our Northampton Road Runners banner and posed, ready for that award-winning shot. A security guard ran across the gallery and, slow motion-like, leapt at us to disrupt the picture just as the photographer was clicking the lens. In an excellent, broken English accent, he informed us that political banners weren't allowed in the Eiffel Tower, and he would have to confiscate it. Although we explained that it was a running club banner, he told us that rules were rules and advised us to go to the ticket booth at the bottom where we could collect it. Sadly, the booth was closed and the banner was never to be seen again.

Beach Running

I started my beach running journey way before the Paris Marathon trip. It was in the final weeks of training for that first Great North Run. We had a week in Spain at my mother-in-law's timeshare apartment, and, not wanting to disrupt my schedule, I took my kit and popped a few runs in during the week. The day we flew home, we immediately drove to Bournemouth for another family weekend, and I did my final training run of 11.5 miles along the promenade. Of course, I went back to do the Bournemouth Half Marathon several times. All these runs were beach heaven.

Now one thing I learned very quickly about running along the coast is, that things that seem close are actually further away than you think. If you pick a landmark, say the pier or the building in the distance, it's probably twice as far as you think.

My first training run in Fuengirola in Spain was hot. I thought to myself, I'll run to that rock at the end of the beach, turn around and run back. Simple. That should be a nice six-mile run. It ended up being nearly nine. Survival expert Bear Grylls said that If you mentally measure the distance of something across the water, double your estimation, and you'll be closer to the correct answer. Big open spaces are bigger than we think, and a great expanse of water can distort our perspective. If you're planning an open water swim, this could be extremely useful to take note of.

A year after Lanza, we headed to the neighbouring island of Fuerteventura for another half marathon running holiday. This was the first time I'd visited the island since the freak accident that led to my brain injury four years earlier, so it was an emotional trip that brought back some painful memories.

The route was in the north of the island and took place in The Parque Natural de las Dunas de Corralejo, which boasts the largest sand dunes in the Canary Islands. The book, *Running Hot & Cold* by Doug Richards, is full of great stories about running in extreme conditions. Doug tells his story of completing the Marathon des Sables, dubbed *The Toughest Footrace on Earth!* It involves running over 150 miles over six days across the Sahara Desert in temperatures exceeding 50 degrees.

The Media Marathon Internacional Dunas de Fuerteventura was more my bag because I was into half marathons and not ultra-events. It was a more manageable thirteen miles of running along rocky sand trails and over sand dunes in the hot October sun with temperatures in the mid-twenties with a slight breeze. At the halfway point, the route made a u-turn taking in its only climb over a small mountain trail before dropping back down a sandy trail. Like the expanse of water giving a false sense of distance measurement, so does a vast desert-like space. On the way back towards the finish, you can see the blue Atlantic Ocean to the right and a large hotel, in view, on the beach. It took three miles before it actually looked any bigger. I couldn't imagine how much tougher the Marathon des Sables would be.

The sand was quite compact, unlike running along a sandy beach where your feet would sink. This was a strange sensation as it was soft, but the top level of the surface would displace slightly, taking just a little extra energy out of the legs. You couldn't even hear footsteps hitting the firm sand beneath your feet.

The finish line was near a little shopping centre called El Campanario. The clock tower on top of one of the buildings became the next focal point to aim for. It's quite unique to see the finish line of a race from such a distance as many events take part in built-up areas. Yet again, those four miles seemed much further than the eye perceived.

This was one of my favourite running experiences ever, being in a place of natural beauty with the distant sound of the sea. It was breath-taking.

Cow Bells, Jeans and Barefoot Runners

Have you ever felt unsuitably dressed for something? Perhaps you arrived at a party in fancy dress only to realise that it was just smart-casual? Maybe you wore a suit and everyone else was dressed casually at a function or, perhaps the other way around?

Earlier in this book, I talked about my early runs in my unbranded black trainers and cotton vest, and, like some of my running friends in their early running days, we've all worn kit that we've felt hasn't been right. However, Jules and I embarked on a backpacking trip to Goa a few years ago, and I just so happened to find out the Goa River Marathon was slap bang in the middle of our trip. And I mean literally! It was on week two and halfway through our loosely planned route through the state.

Jules decided to enter the 10K and I entered the half (of course). I was immediately nervous about the 6:30am start, not because I'm lazy but because I struggle to eat a good breakfast that early. OK, I will admit it, I'm not an early riser, and brain injury plays havoc with fatigue if my body clock goes out of sync. What the hell though? It'll be such an experience. And that was an understatement.

Running in India was incredible. We squeezed in a few final training runs on the beach as the sun set in the weeks before the event. Locals and tourists looked at us as if we'd landed from another planet as they all went about their daily business of working extremely hard or relaxing on the beach.

We arrived for one night only in the Goan city of Vasco Da Gama to prepare for the following day's race. The place was busy, full of the hustle and bustle and very, very hot. After checking into a lovely apartment in the suburbs, we boarded a cramped and smelly bus headed and to the race village to collect our numbers. Named after the Portuguese explorer, Vasco has very little in the form of tourist attractions, so we wandered around for a while looking for somewhere to eat. A local cafe in a small shopping centre proved to be the easiest option but served very basic food to cater for the workers that were flooding in from the nearby shipyard. We returned to the apartment in the afternoon with some basic snacks. Being so far out of the centre, we struggled to find somewhere to eat the night before the race, so we ate the snacks of crisps and bananas while watching the sunset from the balcony. It wasn't the best pre-race meal by a long shot.

The next issue was working out how to get to the start. It was too far to walk, and we had no idea of the bus routes early in the morning. Below the apartment was a spa, and the receptionist lady, who'd held the key to the apartment, offered to book us a taxi. After a quick phone call, she told us the driver would pick us up at 5:45am. Argh, how early?

The following morning, we woke up a little bleary-eyed but dressed in our running kit and headed downstairs. Breakfast consisted of two frozen bananas as the fridge setting was too high and iced our fruit and water. Right on cue, the taxi pulled up outside and the driver took us to the start. He dropped us off a stone's throw from the line and asked us what time we wanted picking up. Having not thought about getting back to the apartment, we made a quick calculation and gave him a time. I pulled out my wallet to pay him and he said, 'No worries, pay me later!' Wow, how trusting.

The pre-race buzz was surreal in the dark. It was total chaos as people moved in every direction. Many runners were dressed in a full running kit of vests, shoes and shorts, as you'd expect to see at a big event. However, many Indian runners wore jeans, t-shirts and trainers, and some were barefoot. It soon became apparent that they were planning to run in that attire as they had their numbers pinned to the front or back. I've never seen so many smiling and excited faces as running a big event is something we take for granted in England, but events are fewer in India.

We both looked for the toilet and asked a guy wearing a high-viz top. He pointed at a wall in the distance and, as we approached, we realised that was his toilet suggestion. I will confess to using the bushes or a tree in the past, but we were on an open cricket field with hundreds of strangers around, and Jules wasn't too keen. We did find the portaloos, thankfully.

My race started at 6:30 am and Jules's was at 8:00am, giving her more time to get nervous. Jules isn't as keen a runner as me, so I was mindful of her being stuck in a strange city, in the dark with lots of people milling around. However, she gave me the usual pre-race hug and off I went.

The route hugged the Zuari River and was around six miles out and back. I settled into a pace in the crowd of people and noticed many Indian runners running in those above-mentioned inappropriate running clothes. I passed a guy wearing jeans and a thick hoodie. At this point, the temperature was approaching 30 degrees, and he already looked very awkward in the first mile. Some others wore traditional Indian headwear and robes and looked glamorous for an early morning run. One thing that was evident was the buzz of the local population. There were many smiles and excited cheers as it was clear that they were probably running their first event. I again realised how much the western culture takes running for granted.

An American runner had settled at the same pace right behind me. He joined in the enthusiastic cheering and whooping and kept repeating the same line, 'Marathon runners, alllllriiiight!' The marathon had started ninety minutes earlier, so the front runners were returning along the opposite side of the road. I knew I needed to either up my pace or slow down because it was now getting irritating.

Now, if you've ever visited Goa, you will realise that you can't walk a couple of hundred metres without seeing a cow, so, without surprise, I found myself navigating my way around many of these sacred animals along the route. They just wander around casually, ignoring the hundreds of people running past. Also on the course were local residents, collecting food and water from the market stalls that lined the river. Men, women and children, laden with goods, carefully hurried across the road, which would probably have been busy with traffic but today had people.

The route became brighter as the sun rose over the river and the colours became richer. I could now see boats chugging along the water as if they were racing us to the turning point.

Still being followed by my American marathon running fan, I suddenly had a lucky break to ditch him. Well, it was actually a little unlucky as my stomach cramped up and my pace dropped. The frozen breakfast banana began to play havoc with my gut, so I went to a portaloo by the side of the road. It seemed about 100 degrees inside and unpleasant, but at least I could no longer hear the marathon mantra.

Thankfully my stomach settled after another quick pit stop, but it left me feeling dehydrated and low on energy. The temperature felt hotter and the air more humid and it became difficult to sweat. I relaxed a little more and just started to enjoy the surroundings of this unique experience. It also gave me time to watch the 10K runners going in the opposite direction as they were now going inland as we returned towards the coast. I ran in the middle of the road, next to the unbroken white line and saw Jules approaching in the distance. She was looking strong and suddenly caught my eye, along with some frantic waving. After a quick mid-race hug, we both carried on.

I crossed the finish line smiling but very low on energy. My running vest was completely stuck to my body and the sweat began to run down my legs. The finish funnel was chaos. It was loud and people were going in every direction, some heading back onto the course to look for friends, as one lone marshal did his best to try and restore order. It was like peeing in the wind, as the saying goes.

A lovely, petite Indian lady hung a finisher medal around my neck and gave me a huge smile saying, 'well done' in broken English. I collected my bag from the chaotic bag collection system and went to a big tent to sit down for a moment. Suddenly a very excited man approached me shouting, 'Sir, you did it. Curry? Beer? You deserve it sir. Please, come!' He gestured towards a massive, long table with another crowd of people talking very loudly. At this point, I really couldn't face a beer and a curry at 8:30 in the morning. I smiled politely, shook his hand and opened my bag to change my top. A minute later, he returned with a portion of curry and said, 'Sir, you look tired, so I get curry for you. Well done sir, you eat!' I was so humbled that I got to my feet to shake hands again and told him I'd eat it in a minute. He gave me the biggest smile and congratulated me another three or four times before heading back into the crowd. Please don't tell him that I didn't eat the curry.

The next task was to somehow watch Jules cross the line. I returned to the finish area's absolute carnage, and it seemed like another thousand or so people had turned up. The noise of chatter and shouting coupled with people going in every direction was almost unbearable. By some amazing stroke of luck, Jules suddenly tapped me on the back. She'd finished a minute before and somehow navigated her way through the crowd and spotted me straight away. She told me that she'd almost bottled the run in the 90 minutes waiting for the start but then loved it. I was delighted. We also later learned that she finished tenth in her age category, which was a remarkable feat.

Now, do you somehow wonder how something that shouldn't work works? We crossed the road and saw a few hundred taxis parked at the side of the road but above the noise behind us we heard the call, 'Hey, Mr Mark, over here sir!' Our driver was waiting and beckoning us to his cab. How he found us is beyond me.

We sunk into the car seats and left the noise behind us as we headed back to the quiet suburban apartment to change and get ready for our trip to the south of Goa. The driver excitedly asked us questions about the run and then offered to take us to our next destination later that afternoon. His friendly customer service and trust landed him the job. We learned all about his family and life as a police officer. Travelling is a real lesson, and, in a short 24 hours, we'd seen a whole new culture and dynamic of the world, not just in running but in life.

Costa Del Running

Us Brits love Spain and holidaying in the many established coastal resorts, perhaps sipping sangria while hearing Viva España playing its cliché tune through the rusting bar speakers. Sun, sea and sand all year round. We'd already headed to the Canary Islands for a race but decided to add more Spanish culture to our running trips.

October is a lovely time for a trip to the island of Majorca. It's much quieter, you can pick up some outstanding deals, plus it's also a little cooler than the hot summer. This makes it ideal to do the Palma Majorca Marathon Festival. Naturally, there's a half marathon option (for me) and a 10K (for Jules). I said that like they'd arranged it especially for us.

After a few days of beach time and lovely food in the resort of Santa Ponsa, we made our way to the island's capital for race day. The start is on the seafront, right in the shadow of the imposing Palma Cathedral. A 10K out and back route hugging the seafront is followed by a winding second half of the race through the narrow city streets. One minute you're running along a road barely wide enough for a car, and then, a quick turn later, you're in a big square with people sipping coffee and eating cake, watching runners speed by. The tall buildings offer shade to fend off the sun that is still hot enough to have an effect.

The route also takes runners right past the cathedral itself, making this part of the race really special. You wind past tourists cheering you on while snapping pictures of this beautiful building. The finish line is also at the same point, albeit back at street level this time. I enjoyed every step of this race, running alongside competitors from various European countries. The marathon route was two laps of the course, but as much as I'd enjoyed it, I was happy enough to cross the finish line and steer away from another lap.

This event was even more special when waiting in the finish pen, as I knew Jules would only be a few minutes away from the line. The 10K had started slightly later than the half, so I tracked her on her phone and saw the dot on the map indicating she was in the last kilometre. Much to the disgust of the spectators and a few finishers, I waited for her yards from the line. A marshal told me to move on, but I smiled, faked a muscle spasm, and pretended to stretch against the barrier next to the spectators. A lady then said a few words, asking me for a second time to move on so she could watch the race. I showed her the blue dot on my phone approaching and explained my wife was close by. She smiled when she understood and joined me in cheering Jules over the line. After my moment of debatable selfishness, there was only one way to celebrate such a lovely run: to drive back to Santa Ponsa, find a restaurant and eat the biggest pizza ever. Thankfully, it was mission accomplished as we sat in the afternoon sun next to the beach, ate pizza, and drank a nice cool beer.

Have you ever been to Benidorm? We decided to take on the next fun challenge in the Costa Blanca party capital. I'd holidayed there when I was 16 and thought it was the greatest place on earth but returning in my forties would give me a different perspective. I'm sure you know someone who's been for a stag or hen party here or perhaps been on one yourself. Maybe you've seen the TV programme Benidorm too. This place is everything it portrays: fun, fun and more fun. It's cheesy, boozy, tacky, and friendly but retains some charm and culture.

We stayed in the old town and took in the sights of the live music bars and tapas restaurants that hug the promenade in the shadow of the towering hotels. It was indeed fun and lively.

Race night was on Saturday at 6:30 pm, meaning you have a whole day to avoid partying and eating badly. We managed to abstain from the above temptations throughout the day and made our way to the start line, Jules doing the 10K and me the half marathon. Yep, the usual pattern. Bon Jovi's Living On A Prayer was booming out of the many speakers lining the rammed start area. The PA announcer bellowed out motivational and promotional words to further build the excitement.

The first part of the race went along the main street for a mile or so before turning back onto the Levante Beach promenade in front of the bars. The atmosphere was electric, with an inebriated crowd cheering like their football team had won the World Cup. It's difficult to keep calm and focused when the buzz and energy are so charged. If we thought that part was loud, the old town was louder. The high buildings captured the noise and dumped it back onto the running crowd. Benidorm was like a running party.

Suddenly the route left the old town and headed along much quieter Poniente Beach. The noise was still ringing in my ears, but the peace was surreal. After a couple of miles, the route headed away from the sea and up a short climb known as the Highway to Hell. Here stood a mad guy wearing a wig and playing a fake, inflatable guitar as AC/DC blasted out of the speakers. I was in my element with the music but also knocked slightly off-balance every time I passed a speaker at ear height.

The half marathon was two laps of the same course, and, bizarrely, the crowds that were evident on the first lap had dispersed a little, giving yet another dimension to this amazing race atmosphere. The Highway to Hell man was still going strong about 45 minutes later though, this time rocking out to Sweet Child o' Mine from Guns N' Roses. Brilliant!

As Benidorm's partygoers had moved elsewhere, finishing the race in the evening was brilliant. We returned to our hotel for food at the restaurant before indulging in a celebratory beer. After completing the 10K, Jules declared her love of running but only in other countries.

We loved the Beni experience and vowed to return to do it again. Strangely, a few weeks after the event, the whole world went into lockdown with the pandemic. Benidorm was the last place we'd visited pre-pandemic and not being able to travel left us with heavy hearts. We longed to get our passports out and begin our wanderlust again. Jules and I even watched Benidorm on Netflix over and over to try and capture that fun memory.

Thankfully, we were lining the streets again for our second go at the event two years on. This time, there was a new route but it still included plenty of promenades and the old town to experience the noise. The first couple of miles ran along Levante Beach again and it was bedlam. Like before, partygoers were going bonkers at everyone running past, making your stride a little bit quicker. After leaving the seafront, we got to run towards Benidorm Palace, famous for its live entertainment shows. About five miles into the route, it passed along a strip of bars in the new town. I managed to watch about five minutes of a football match, passing the big screens in the bars and was also offered a combined total of around 30 bottles of beer from different party animals. As much as beer was tempting, I declined. The support was amazing. Jules later told me that she ran this stretch with Spiderman too!

After passing through the noisy old town, the 10K route now peeled back to the start-finish, so we were just left with half marathon runners. We headed out and back along the quieter Poniente Beach. Sadly, there was no Highway to Hell man this time, although that meant no hill to climb.

At the turning point, I looked back and saw the end of Levante Beach, knowing we had to re-navigate our way back there before another about-turn to the finish line. The focal point was a hotel shaped like a K. K for Kennedy; I kept thinking! It seemed to take an age to reach. Remember the distorted perception of fixed points when looking across the water? Once I'd reached this, there were a couple of miles left of the course. It was amusing running along the main road through the town and passing a speed limit sign telling runners they were breaking the 10km/h limit. Sadistically I sped up to try and get a reading of 20km/h but didn't quite make it.

Medals, T-shirts and Goodies
Benidorm running part two was just as special as part one. Jules was cheering at the finish as I made my final few steps towards the finish line and collected my goodie bag and medal. Having run many events, I have a cupboard full of t-shirts and a box full of medals which are fond treasures.

I rummaged through my goodie bag at Beni, firstly looking for a bottle of water and immediately downed it. We made our way to a nearby bar for a sit-down and a beer, of course! The next exciting bit was to see what else was in the bag. After finding the standard leaflets advertising races and running gear and a few chocolate bars, I discovered some t-bags and a bag of white powder. I asked the lady behind the bar what it was, and she told me it was salt! Yes, that's right, a kilogram of salt. Now, I've had some post-race gifts in my time, but salt has to be the most bizarre one to date. The bar staff gratefully accepted the gift of a couple of kilos of salt. I was thankful as it would've weighed too much for our hand luggage on the return flight and customs might've mistaken it for something more sinister too.

———

Stories From the Field - Real Life Runners and Goodie Bags
The goodie bag can contain some lovely souvenirs, but there are also some random things. Andy said, '*I got a rather splendid towel at a Bedford Harriers race with their club emblem on the towel.*' *That did remind me of their well-thought-out gifts each time I've done it. One year, runners were awarded a drawstring rucksack bag too.*'

A favourite race of our club is the Colworth Marathon Challenge. There are three races making up a marathon distance over the weekend. My running mate Darren reminded me of a few of the gifts in the past, '*The shot glasses from Colworth are up there in terms of weird gifts. Don't forget the beer towel one year too. Every event, they give you as much iced tea you could drink.*'

Jo got a lovely loaf of bread from a big bakery at a local 5K which made her enter the following year again. She was disappointed that the delicious gift wasn't repeated though.

In the 'not so delicious category', Paula said, '*I had a kilo bag of rice once, I believe it was in the goody bag pre-London Marathon one year*' and Zoe said, '*When I did the Benidorm Half, I got a 250ml carton of fish sauce!*' Hmm, there must be a random theme at Benidorm here, that would go well with the huge bag of salt maybe! Packets of dried pasta were also mentioned quite a lot, but one person said they were given a cabbage when they crossed the line. Now, this is starting to sound weird.

Christopher got a packet of soup at Torremolinos, but the organisers were redeemed by adding a fleece, beach towel, and a medal.

Neil said, '*I did the Birmingham Black Country Half. I got a stick of rock, like seaside candy rock! It's still in in a drawer four years later. Birmingham isn't that close to the sea, making it even more random!*'

I was chatting to Daniel after a parkrun one day and he told me, '*One odd one was some mint-flavoured caffeine chewing gum. It tasted awful!*'

Chris from Parklands Jog and Run said, '*I was given a 20-kilogram sack of potatoes for doing the Flitton Potato Race.*' Quite an apt gift, I guess. He continued, '*I got some 'She Wees' once at Twilight Run, and I won a gas mask for first place at World War Run!*' I'm going to be completely honest, I didn't know what She Wees were until a quick internet search enlightened me.

Michelle, my friend who runs a brilliant fitness group called Step Forward with Lewis shared, '*My favourite has been beer at a New Orleans 5K. That was the first time after a race I got one, but it seems to be the in thing now.*' That is very true, I've been presented with bottles of beer post-race too.

Guy said he was given an ashtray after a 10-mile race in the nineties. Now that is probably something you wouldn't get nowadays and not something I'd want, being a non-smoker. How strange indeed.

––––

Thoughts Running Through the Mind

Travel and running are two passions I've managed to combine well. The more you enjoy something, the more likely you are to carry out the task. Some of my favourite training sessions are the ones where we have loads of fun and encourage each other.

The thoughts in this chapter are simple. What could you hook together for double enjoyment? Perhaps you have a hobby that could involve family or friends or something that combines fitness and fun?

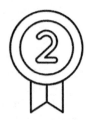

10. Second Best

Are you competitive? I'm not! I've never had that absolute will to win and be the best; I just want to do my best and not worry about others. Winning massively gives me imposter syndrome. Don't get me wrong, I love getting all the correct answers in a music quiz or being champion at Monopoly from time to time, but sport is a different matter.

Being a quiet and shy kid at school, being popular and winning were two things that went hand in hand, or so it seemed. I did neither! My final three years of state school education were spent at Northampton School for Boys and being around hundreds of lads every day was a cocktail of high testosterone and competitive spirit from the minute you arrived until the minute you went home. I was happy to sit in the background and be a spectator for the most part. At times it was funny but other times, it could be a little intimidating.

There was always competition to be the funniest, loudest, most quick-witted, strongest and fastest but never the most academic. There was one bizarre competition to see who could push through the doors into or out of the tuck shop area, and this so-called pastime resembled a ruck in rugby. For no apparent reason, a couple of lads would be going one way and some the other. Instead of politely saying '*after you*', they'd push against each other until someone started *winning*. The watching crowd would join in and start pushing out of the door, whereas the other lads trying to enter would push from the other side of the threshold. It would be like a reverse tug o' war until one side of the crowd subsided and the other successfully got through the double doorway. There would be huge cheers from the winners, and everyone would go on with their day. Yeah, I know, I'm typing this and wondering what the point was too, but it never stopped me from occasionally joining in. I guess that's what lads do!

One day, my mate, Norman, talked me into entering a Friday lunchtime competition called Champion Athlete. It was a decathlon-style challenge with one weekly event combining track and field events. I may have been shy, but I've always been open-minded and like to make impulse decisions. Norman was a very academic student but also excellent at rugby, and, as the school was rugby mad, I guess I was protected from bullying because I was his mate. I'm always grateful to Norman for that and he used to let me copy his homework from time to time.

Naturally, some of the sports stars from the school signed up for Champion Athlete, including a few troublemakers. I guess it was a welcome relief from the competition of who could throw their school bag (or someone else's) the furthest down the hill on the school field. Yep, that was another pastime at our school too.

With the 100 metres and the javelin out of the way, I'd also completed the 400-metre hurdles, very badly. Next was the shot-put. At age 14, I probably weighed about nine stone and was quite wiry in my build (or skinny as some people called me). I certainly wasn't built for throwing things, especially heavy items. Even the javelin wasn't a huge success, but now I had to coordinate a heavy cannonball, coupled with spinning around a few times and hurling it as far as it would go. As you can guess, it didn't go far.

One of the sporty troublemakers had mocked me for my previous three efforts and now decided to step it up a notch. I was sitting in last place and well behind the next competitor, who also received a bit of ridicule. Most of the time, I would walk away, find some solace somewhere quiet and ignore these comments as fighting and confrontation were things I couldn't handle (and still can't). However, this time I decided to stand up for myself and just asked the guy to be kind for once and support everyone for having a go. Thinking the teacher would be on my side and a few of the lads in the competition would too, I waited for the response. Naturally, my mate Norman agreed, but everyone else fell silent. The teacher shrugged his shoulders and set up the next competitor to throw.

As we headed back to the changing room, I tried again to reason with a small group and the teachers, but, again, it fell on deaf ears. In the changing room, the said mocking lad grabbed my can of drink from my lunch and downed it in one go before handing me the empty can. I got changed, announced I was quitting and walked out.

On the flip side of the coin, the school also had a togetherness spirit. For every fellow student who would mock you, there was one who would encourage you. I was fortunate to be in a form group that remained together throughout our three years at the school. We were the Q group in the third year, known as 3Q. Moving up to the fourth year, we became 4Q. Our teacher, Mr Turner, walked in on our first day and said, 'Four-que, that's unfortunate!' You may need to read this out loud a few times, but not in front of any kids! Amazingly, none of us got it straight away.

Anyhow, the Q Class were good lads, and we never really excelled at interclass competitions, so we dug in like underdogs and had a go at everything. Our drama play at Christmas was a disaster. It was called 'When Santa Claus Meets St Trinians'. However, we had great fun writing and performing it. Aside from Norman, we didn't have any rugby stars but put up a spirited show in the rugby tournament. On sports days, we cheered each other on, no matter where anyone finished in events. I guess this encouraged me just to take part in stuff and not worry about winning.

Fast forward to my running days, and that became an immediate love of the sport. Suddenly, I'd found something that I was reasonable at, and I didn't feel that I needed to win. Racking up PBs was precisely what it stood for, a personal best! You could simply be your best self and not worry about others around you.

In my first races, people commented on how good my times were. I was pleased with a 5K in less than 23 minutes, my Silverstone 10K in less than 48 minutes and a half marathon of sub-two hours at the Great North Run. I was finishing around halfway in the field in most races, and that suited me. I was the middle-of-the-road kid at school, and now I could be in the middle-of-the-running pack. That fitted my laid-back approach to life in general.

One evening, I entered a fun run at my local park and came third. It was an untimed event with a basic marked-out course, but I began to think about what it would feel like to win a race. Just once, it would be great to stand on the podium and celebrate a gold medal of sorts. It wasn't a huge goal of mine but something to ponder. I had no desire to be the athlete who dedicated every moment to training and conditioning that would be needed to run that one-hour half marathon, so I continued enjoying my running.

First by Miles
Winning and not feeling worthy is a case of the good old imposter syndrome rearing its head again. Yep, it knows how to dilute your moment of glory at the best of times.

There was King of the Hill at the Moulton Fun Run that I mentioned earlier. I was relaxed about winning that one because I didn't win the race, although I was gutted all the same.

A couple of years before, I did cross the line with my arms in the air and not quite knowing how to celebrate. I'd done it, I'd won my first race. It was the Parklands Jog and Run Halloween Mile. After the 30 competitors had crossed the line, I was presented with a framed certificate, and a quick photo was snapped on a phone camera. That was it, finally a first-place finish.

A good mate of mine, Chris, runs a brilliant local running group called Parklands Jog and Run. He'd introduced me to interval training, which sounds serious, but I found to be enjoyable. Chris is a top local runner who has been winning track events for years and then turned his hand to obstacle racing, winning those events too. He's now a Vet's Master on the track. However, like most excellent runners, he was one of the humblest and encouraging people ever, not arrogantly celebrating his own achievements but helping others begin and improve their running journeys. He also sets up fun events under the umbrella of Quirky Races.

For Halloween, he set up an event called the Halloween Mile, so I entered. It was two laps around the field in the dark and volunteers jump out to scare you. I ran it in just under six and a half minutes, and then Chris presented me with the certificate at the end. That was it, my glittering running career now had a first-place finish on its CV. Of course, I laughed at the end. It was a fun run with no competitive weight to it, so I felt imposter syndrome at coming first. I was also under-dressed, wearing a regular running kit as I was on my way to my running club for a five-mile run.

That did get me wondering how I could finish first in a competitive event. As good as it would be, my uncompetitive side would kick in, and I would play it down further. I'd probably be too polite and let the runner behind me finish first while clapping them over the line.

Chris hosted one-mile time trails and more fun runs at his Parklands group. These were always great fun as I became good friends with a fellow runner called Mick, who was a few years older than me. I was immediately drawn to his funny, quick-witted banter and the ability to poke fun and offend people without offending them.

Not only is Mick really encouraging, but he's super competitive, and we began to egg each other on at parkruns. It was a fun, light-hearted battle between the two of us and another one of my club buddies, Pete. We were always full of congratulations for whoever finished ahead that day. It was good-spirited competition which Mick certainly got more pleasure from winning than Pete and I did.

I did have another Parklands victory under my belt at a Christmas Mile Fun Run, beating Mick home that day. I can still picture his face when Chris presented me with a winner's medal this time. Mick clapped while hurling some friendly, expletive abuse in my direction. What surprised me most was that I'd been out with some friends the night before and had a bit of a long-overdue reunion. My body wasn't accustomed to drinking the amount of alcohol that we did in our teens and early twenties, so is it fair to say that I was a little tender? Thankfully, the Christmas run took place in the early afternoon, allowing me a little recovery time.

After my 15 in 2015, I took a little break from racing for a few months. The Thailand trip was great, but I was fearful of the collapsed lung, and my anxiety was relatively high, although, at the time, I didn't realise it. I started researching the after-effects of brain injury and what I could do to eradicate some of these foggy feelings. Then I'd become a bit paranoid, thinking that perhaps it's better not to know this information. For example, if someone says, if you sprint for a minute, you might develop a headache, then you're more likely to get a headache after 60 seconds of effort. OK, that's complete nonsense and a pretty naff example, but you get the idea that if you put a thought into someone's head, they'll probably believe it.

Everything about brain injury still centred on one major topic: fatigue. Of course, I could write a whole book on many other side effects (well, we actually did – What The Hell Just Happened?), but fatigue was the primary factor. If you're fatigued, it affects your concentration, mood, memory, ability to walk in a straight line, or string a sentence together and a whole host of other things. It sounds like being drunk, doesn't it?

Fatigue and tired shouldn't be confused too! Tired isn't good but can generally be managed by regulating your body clock. Adults need between seven and nine hours of sleep on average, which needs to be practised seven days a week. If you've ever had jet lag, you'll know that your body clock will become accustomed to the new time zone a couple of days later. Fatigue doesn't work like that.

Brain injury fatigue can be debilitating, and it wipes me out. It can also hit when least expected. Background noise, flashing lights, multiple conversations, lots of information, filling in forms or answering questions are all things that can cause me to feel fatigued suddenly. This could also happen after a great night's sleep and could happen at ten o'clock in the morning. People will say things like, '*Oh, it's OK, I'm tired too*' or '*you just need to go to bed earlier*' as well as the classic, '*How come you're tired when you got up late this morning and slept this afternoon too?*'. I won't mention the all-time classic, '*it's your age!*' Oh, hang on, I just did! Over time, I've become relatively passive about these statements because most people who say them mean well and display empathy. If any of my friends are reading this, honestly, you haven't offended me.

At this point in my life, I didn't understand this. I was still in the mindset that fatigue would start to ease, my memory would go back to what it was, and I would return to the person I once was. However, research online says brain injury sufferers may never recover fully, and these symptoms will last forever. Most recovery occurs in the first six months to a year, and the scars left will heal much slower. Here I am talking of brain injury, but this also applies to many other injuries and illnesses. Cancer treatment after-effects certainly still affect Jules today too.

My first round of research took place in Lanzarote on a beautiful sunny afternoon while lying by the pool. Usually, our holidays are pretty get up and go and explore but running the half marathon and the silly bike ride was adventurous enough for us on that trip. I decided to try making things easier and opted for more afternoon naps on days between travelling up and down the country. Taking the train instead of the car seemed a much more sensible option as driving was just wiping me out more than ever. As much as I didn't want to, I decided not to race for a couple of months and stop pushing for PBs. It was tough to make this choice because running gave me such a high, but I'd also read about the boom-and-bust cycle. The enforced break due to my second collapsed lung also took that decision out of my hands for a little longer. After not running for a few weeks, I eased myself back into just being involved in doing my local parkrun and then running short distances on club nights and slowing down my pace.

Honestly, I don't remember much about this period of my life, as anxiety and brain injury combined tend to block things out, and the sense of time becomes a little warped. I do remember being quite withdrawn at times and avoiding busy situations. When I was in school, I'd deliver my workshop and find an excuse to get off-site as soon as possible. Going to a quiet cafe or even a supermarket and sitting in the car eating lunch was more appealing than the crowded and busy staffroom. I just didn't want information overload from conversations. Despite these changes, I was still powering through, and, in all truth, probably not sticking to my intentions.

We're all guilty of trying to create a new habit but then realising that a few months have passed, and you haven't actually started yet. I have friends who are constantly joining gyms and paying money for a membership which only satisfies the gym's bank account. You must push through a conscious pain barrier to create a new habit. It may be painful and uncomfortable at first but the rewards will follow later.

Running is an excellent example of this. A beginner will have great intentions but then will have to deal with all those things outside one's comfort zone. We talked about loads of them in the Beginner's Guide chapter. Not being quick enough, worrying about what people think and suchlike. Once the beginner gets out of the door, they must feel the pain of using new muscles that will ache and quickly be out of breath if they haven't engaged in exercise for a while. Ouch, the following day, they have discovered muscles they didn't know they had or reappear like a long-lost friend who hasn't been in touch for some time. This is when many may quit. It's much more comfortable to sit back on the sofa and return to the same thoughts and feelings. I'm sure that creating a positive habit is much harder than continuing a negative one.

Anyway, I'm goal-driven! I didn't fully understand brain injury and was often told I'd be fine. Even the hospital would say to me that on my annual visits. Headway told me it was normal to experience these things, so on I went. For most of my life, things always seem to work out through positivity, so let's get back to winning a race.

I came across a local 10K in the village of Earls Barton and posted it in our running club Facebook group. The run was part of a village festival on a Sunday afternoon and seemed relaxed. I have several friends in the village, so I entered and thought it would be ideal to run and catch up with them. After realising that none of my club mates would be running, this seemed like a good day for a record attempt. OK, I don't go to races to try and win, but after collecting my number and surveying the field, it looked like there weren't any other club runners there. Following a short race briefing, the organiser urged us to the start line, but the field of runners was quite reluctant, saying they weren't quick enough for that. Three of us broke clear as the starting gun sounded. Yes, the starter actually fired a pistol, how wonderful! As we rounded the village cricket pitch, one guy said, 'balls to this' and started to drop back as he realised the pace was too quick. Unfortunately for me, the other chap began to pull clear. Undeterred, I gave chase as we headed out into the countryside and towards a local country park. He started to disappear into the distance and showed no signs of slowing down. I wondered if he might get lost, but it was unlikely as the course looped around a reservoir. By the time I'd completed the lap of the water, he was nowhere in sight. I turned back onto the country road to complete the last mile cross the line in second. The winner was three minutes ahead and took his award in a mini presentation, but before, the announcer said, '...and in second place with a strong run, Mark Kennedy of Northampton Road Runners!' Brilliant, it was a proud moment. Of course, I had the moment of imposter syndrome and looked for every reason to play it down at first, but I soon realised it was a fantastic achievement and was bursting with excitement.

I did go back to the same event the following year and secretly hoped that none of my quick club mates would read my post on the club's Facebook page. They didn't, but three runners were faster than me, so I was fourth this time. The event victory was still elusive, so the Parklands Halloween certificate and the Christmas Fun Run were going to be my proud moments.

Before my mini-break from running, I also managed a second-place finish at Hackworth parkrun on Christmas Day. It's a challenging course of three laps which involved a zigzag climb up a hill before a quick descent and then a muddy grass section. Well, it was muddy in December anyway. I led the course for one and a half laps before a chap whizzed past me on the downhill section and then pulled out of sight. Like the Earls Barton 10K, I was proud of this. Finishing second in a parkrun is quite an achievement when you look at the quality of the times recorded at each venue.

Chapter eight was about personal bests, so perhaps second-place finishes in a 10K and a parkrun and the three one-mile victories in the Parklands Jog and Run events would be fine in my glittering running career as it was unfolding month by month and year by year. Like many other runners, I collected wonderful stories and memories while being part of challenges and seeing others take steps along their journeys. The age-old phrase, *it's not the winning, it's the taking part that counts*, could be used in running. It's a bit of a cliché though. However, it's a mass participation sport where you can compete with yourself if you wish or, perhaps, not even compete at all.

This was a world away from my school days where everything seemed like a competition, and I loved to plod. One evening, I was at the football, watching Northampton Town play in a midweek game. I was chatting to the chap next to me, and he then pointed out that I hadn't remembered him from school. Suddenly the penny dropped, and I remembered being good friends with him, and he instantly became recognisable. One of the things that stuck in my mind was that he was a pretty good footballer and runner and was always encouraging in the inter-class sports tournaments we used to have. He said that he'd heard about my running pursuits and was impressed. We talked about my sporting ability back then, and he said, '*You may think you used to be rubbish at sports at school, but now you'll beat 99% of the lads who were there. We're all too lazy now. Fair play to you mate, amazing!*'

It was heartening to hear those words that summed up not only running but the whole idea of living your life on your own terms. Why should it matter if you finish first, middle or last? He reminded me of the old cross-country days and when he used to finish second to a phenomenal runner called Adharanand Finn. Adharanand, author of the best-selling book, *Running with the Kenyans*, would lead the field by a country mile and nobody could get near him. He was another extremely talented person who would encourage everyone. Even though he was the best, I found him encouraging at whatever sport we were involved in together, whether it was kicking a football at break time or engaging in class competition.

———

Stories From the Field - Real Life Runners and Affirmations

We may not win races, but isn't getting to the finish line a personal victory? Mindset is one of the most significant factors in success with anything in life. Positive self-talk is powerful when creating a positive, growth mindset, so why not create an affirmation to help you get closer to your goal?

Also, I've run many events with a song repeating in my head. Sometimes it's a song I love, and sometimes it's an annoying one. Sometimes it could just be one verse where I suddenly become aware of the lyrics and then realise that my feet are pounding to the beat or the words are uplifting and motivating. One that immediately springs to mind is, *Take It Easy* by *Eagles*. For some reason, it would always pop into my head. I love that song and the band, it's one of many numbers that's kept me going to finish races.

I also remember doing various events where affirmations and positive quotes are painted on signs around the course. These help to lighten the mood and make you smile, but the phrases can impact your performance.

'*Effort doesn't get easier; you just get stronger*', is one of my favourites.

Sadly, due to copywriting laws, we authors aren't allowed to republish song lyrics in our books without permission, so I decided to play it safe and asked runners what their running mantras are. Here are 12 favourites that were shared:

- Run the mile you're in. Right now, it might be tough; the next mile could be faster, easier, or downhill. Just run the mile you're in.
- You started, so you might as well finish.
- I am looking forward to the stairs tomorrow.
- It's just one foot in front of the other and repeat.
- If you finish, you get cake.
- Pain is just weakness leaving the body.
- It's better to finish last than never have the courage to start.
- It's not a race; it's a run.
- It's only a slope (*about hills*).
- Only a parkrun left to go (*with 3.1 miles to go in a long race*).
- Effort doesn't get easier; you just get stronger.
- The faster you run, the sooner you rum (*haha*).

———

Thoughts Running Through the Mind

As mentioned above, positive self-talk greatly affects your performance at anything in life. Henry Ford once said, '*If you think you can or you think you can't, you're right!*' Wow, it's spot on really, if you think you can't do something, the chances are, you probably won't.

I meet many people who say they can't run to the end of the street, and sadly they're also right. They can't because they won't.

Again, think about what your goals are and then think about how you can achieve them. If you ask yourself a question like, '*How can I run a mile?*' your mind will immediately start thinking of ideas and options.

Mr Ford was successful in the motor business on his own, creating growth mindsets allowing him to achieve his goals and dreams. He believed he could and focused on that word 'can' throughout his life.

Your challenge is to find out ways to turn the *I can't* into *I can*.

'*I can't*', '*I won't*' and '*I don't know*' are all phrases that will stop your brain's processes in its tracks. Every time you say these words, change your language to, '*How can I?*', '*I could*' or '*I will*' and '*What could the answer be?*'

The second thought is around music. A tune can be a powerful and uplifting motivator to help you daily. I have so many playlists (including the Eagles, of course) that help me feel energised for various activities and tasks, just as a mood lifter or even memory jogger.

Why not create a playlist of your favourite tunes to get you jumping around and ready to take on your next challenge?

If you go to Half Man, Half Marathon on Spotify, you'll find some of my playlists. I hope you enjoy them.

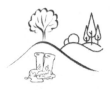

11. Mud, Glorious Mud (and Hills)

In the chapter, Running Into the Wind, there were plenty of analogies about sailing your ship into a storm and surviving. I also talked briefly about life throwing brown stuff at you at times but how I love cross country racing and events like the Grizzly. Well, my life continued to follow a similar path of blurry moments, fatigue and confusion. It was the same old, same old on that front. I asked myself should I continue with this chapter, or will it be too samey as the last ones? OK, let's give it a go! The trouble with anxiety is that it can loop around and won't change until you become a master of it. Mastering anxiety, well, is that possible? Add in a neurological condition, and that's, well, a big brown poo storm! Throw in the fact that I had no bloody idea what was going on in my head, that made it even more confusing. Oh yeah, did I mention that my lack of awareness of these things was also escaping me? I might have even written about this before in an earlier chapter, and I make no apologies about that. I can sometimes repeat myself. I've asked my editor to leave this bit in if I have because I'm totally cool with the neuro-uniqueness in my world now.

I'd experimented with taking some time out of racing like a madman and trying to see if that would take some of the fatigue away. In all honesty, it didn't really work. Coming second in the Earls Barton 10K made me hungry for more. A few days after this race, I came close to my 10K PB at Silverstone, home of the British Grand Prix and my 10K PB and former half marathon PB. Yeah, I reckon it's more famously known for running in my household than F1 racing. OK, stop Mark... that's your wild imagination and neuro-weirdness, as you so eloquently put it.

Another week passed, and I equalled my six-mile PB at Rugby, which was famous for the sport of... yep, Rugby. Life was full of confusion, but I could run. I could run fast, and the East Midlands Grand Prix Series was the ideal place to do it. The EMGP, as it's known for short, is a series of eight races between five miles and 10K. Your best five places count towards a grade in the series; the more you do, the better your chances. As with anything in running, you can compete against yourself or just rock up at one event and enjoy that with no pressure. Amazing!

I did the Banbury 5 and smashed my five-mile PB! It's also worth mentioning Banbury is famous for the Banbury Cross, mentioned in the much-loved 1700s nursery rhyme, Ride a cockhorse to Banbury Cross.

Race, race, race. I'm missing half marathons, so the following weekend, I did the Market Harborough Half on a hot June day. The hill at mile eleven was energy-sapping, and I had nothing left at the finish, but there was no time to stop; half marathon number 64 was ticked off. A few days later, the Harborough 5 (mile) was another series race.

OK, pause for a while. Phew, I need a rest from writing just thinking about this. Three races in a week, and I'm pushing myself at all of them. Market Harborough is famous for being a market town and retains a lovely character. It's only a short drive from Northampton, so a midweek trip was too good to miss. In the race, I was flying and felt like I glided around the course. When I crossed the line, I checked my watch and it read 32:55. This was one second quicker than Banbury the week before. The issue I had now was the wait in anticipation for this to be confirmed. The series didn't publish instant results then, so we had to wait until the following day to find out the confirmed times. Thankfully it matched my watch, and it was another PB.

Despite trying to slow down life in general, I was running to escape. The buzz of pushing for a time was likened to numbing the pain, but the pain I was experiencing was actually the sense of numbness. Running was becoming my escape from the fog. The fog was putting me into a numb state, and it was stuck on a loop. There were times when I felt like crying would've done me the world of good, but I couldn't express much feeling. I'd been into a school and motivated a group of teens but wished the day away so I could get on the train and sit quietly, not having to talk to anyone. Racing still gave me the escape of feeling great, doing something I loved but not having to speak to many people. When running flat out, it's difficult to maintain a conversation of course.

Half marathon numbers 65 and 66 were completed at Adderbury and Northampton, and I recorded good times. Then we headed to Fuerteventura for the magical run across the sand dunes. That was it for longer runs as I scaled back again, doing parkruns and the Three Counties Cross Country Series. The first event was back to Wing and that muddy stream crossing. Thankfully the cows weren't in the field next to the water, so it was only mud we had to wade through on this one.

Talking of mud, this particular year had been a bit muddy, to say the least. As much as I loved running muddy trails, I didn't like the brown stuff in everyday life. Workwise, things became a little strained with the company I was in partnership with. I began making mistakes, like getting teachers' names wrong and even delivering the wrong programme at one school. A couple of schools had also fed back that my session lacked energy. At the time, I didn't understand why but it makes sense now that I lacked energy due to the horrendous fatigue. The partnership with that company ended as the year drew to a close and I was gutted. It hurt and I felt a numb feeling again.

However, Jules was excited as we now had a world of opportunity ahead of us. She was encouraging and saw the chance to stamp our own brand on our business. We could run it on our own terms and create some exciting new ventures. Now, I'm an extremely positive person, but I felt weak with anxiety and battered like a boxer who'd just been floored in the ring. My confidence felt at an all-time low, and my self-esteem was even lower. The timing for a break couldn't have been better as we set off on another backpacking adventure around Southeast Asia, visiting Thailand and Malaysia. It was wonderful! The people, the places and the experience of a different life were magical. We've worked in education and personal development for years and are always big advocates of how much you learn by travelling. Seeing the world as a big place means understanding cultures and how things work in other countries. For example, getting a ferry in Thailand is an experience. We bought a ticket from a travel agent, who then issued us a voucher. The voucher had to be exchanged for a ticket when we boarded a minibus to the ferry port. At the ferry port, the ticket was exchanged for another ticket for the ferry, and we were told to go and buy a pier ticket. Yes, you must pay to get on the pier in order to board the speedboat at the end of the pier. It's impossible to avoid this extra charge. When you have the pier ticket and the ferry ticket, you can now walk along the pier to the desk, where you check onto the speedboat. At this point, your passport is checked as you take the ferry from the Thai mainland to the Thai island. There is no passing of international waters. On the island, you show your passport and ticket again and wait for a long-tail boat to take you from a floating pier to the sand. It's a strange, overly complicated system that just about works, but everyone does it with a smile. The Thai authorities want to employ as many of their country's people as possible so that jobs with processes are created. It's a fascinating learning experience.

Those Muddy Hills

This chapter is called Mud, Mud, Glorious Mud, but we walked a lot of sandy beaches on our backpacking adventure, so you may excuse me if I'm going off track from mud to sandy beaches and Thai boat trips and may think it's my neuro weirdness. However, after flying back from Bangkok, we arrived midweek, so there was no parkrun dash, like our last trip. That didn't mean there was no mad rush though. We landed at London Heathrow, got the train home, slept, got up and then hopped on a train to Manchester for a trip we'd planned for Jules's birthday. After a couple of days in Manchester, we got the train home, slept and then got up the following morning to drive to Norwich for a school gig before returning home for a rest. So much for taking the pressure off.

Where's the mud? Come on, get to the mud I hear you cry! Well, that's what's coming next. After the Norwich gig, there was only a few days rest before I drove to Leicestershire for the Charnwood Hills Fell Race.

The organisers, Bowline Climbing Club, certainly know how to put on a challenging route. This was the third time I'd entered and lined up at the start on a cold February morning. The route of 14 miles fitted into my half marathon category, and I was excited to start my quest for the next target of reaching 75. As the race began, my 68th was underway. A run around a muddy school field allowed the runners to filter out before an orderly queue formed in the bottom corner, where a narrow, muddy lane took everyone out into the fields. A little slope of around five steps caught a few excited runners out, and some had mud on their backsides within the first mile.

I'd seen a little rain on our Asian adventure and had missed the epic downpours in England while we were on the other side of the world. Rain plus fields equals mud, and lots of it! The first couple of miles of this race were reasonably flat and circumnavigated farm fields that were sticky. Next came Bradgate Country Park, which was stunning and has Bradgate House slap bang in the middle and deer roaming free on the grounds. The route took us along the side of the house, which involved navigating narrow trails with tufts of grass, deep ruts and streams to cross. It was an adventure in itself. Old John Tower was also a famous landmark that can be seen for miles. This folly sits on top of the highest point of the park and is shaped like a beer tankard, giving another unofficial name of Old John's Tankard. The myth is the folly was built in honour of a beer-loving miller who was killed in the park. This isn't true, of course, but it's a lovely myth. It was a treat to run up the steep hill and through the folly before descending back down the other side. The rugged landscape made the run so interesting, with plenty of scenery to take in. Many runners will curse a hill because of the difficulty, but the views at the top are magnificent.

I've also done a similar race called the Ridgeway 15K. This goes from Tring in Hertfordshire and is known as one of Britain's oldest roads. The view from the top of the ridge is stunning and takes your mind off the aching quads that have just propelled you to the top. Running through woodland is one of my favourite things ever, and I mean ever - honest! The Ridgeway has a stretch of a few miles beneath the canopy of trees, with views over miles and miles of green fields below.

Back in the Charnwood region, after leaving Bradgate Park, there was another climb that was almost impossible to run up, so putting your hands on your quads while climbing is a good option to get to the top, making sure to glance at the views on the way. I'm not 100% familiar with the area, but while checking an Ordnance Survey Map on the Bowline site, I've seen references to Hunt's Hill, Warren Hill, Ling Hill, Broombrigg Hill and Beacon Hill, to mention a few. Now it's clear where the name Charnwood Hills comes from. The route goes out towards Beacon Hill Country Park before a loop around it, with a hill climb of course, and then retraces its way back again. One random part goes through Lingdale Golf Club, with a few hardcore golfers out for a winter round. They look bemused as muddy runners pass one of the fairways, slipping and sliding everywhere in the mud. After the golf course comes another hill, surprisingly enough. It was so muddy that it was just about possible to stay upright. Every time I planted my feet, they slid one way or the other. A fellow runner somehow ran past me as I was laughing uncontrollably, trying to stay upright and avoid looking like Bambi on ice. He then slid wildly to the left and ended up on his backside. As he climbed to his feet, he looked back to check that I hadn't noticed. Of course, I had, but pretended I hadn't as not to not embarrass him. Honestly, I don't think he actually cared as he continued on his slippery adventure.

Charnwood can only be described as energy-sapping, muddy and sticky. I've hit what's known as the wall in pretty much every marathon I've run. The wall just takes every ounce of your energy away from you, and all you want to do is sit down on the floor and quit. I hit the Charnwood Wall at mile eleven. Urgh! With three miles of a 14-mile race in such beautiful surroundings left, I felt gutted. There is nothing wrong with walking in a race, but I didn't want to walk the final stretch. It was time for the run-walk tactic with a bit of slipping and sliding and trying not to fall over. I stumbled through the rough terrain of Bradgate again, and thankfully, we had no Old John to climb on the way back. My feet went through some knee-deep puddles, but I kept my balance. The final big field was so muddy and sticky that it was like running through treacle. By now, fellow runners were gliding past, or so it seemed. Turning the corner, the last challenge was to climb that little slope onto the school field, but things weren't easy as they appeared. The marshal called out a cry of encouragement as I approached. I smiled, thanked him and built-up what speed I could to make the few steps up the slope. Halfway up, it was like someone pulling the rug from underneath me and I slid straight back down. Picking myself up off all fours, I went for attempt number two but ended up with exactly the same outcome. Another runner went past me as my third effort ended with me sliding back down on all fours. At this point, I was laughing uncontrollably as the marshal put out his hand to pull me up for the fourth try. We did it! Teamwork makes dreams work, and, despite nearly pulling him down the slippery slope with me, I offered him my thanks and wobbled my way to the finish line, still tittering away to myself. I was shattered as I walked back to the school gym to collect my bag. These races don't have medals or t-shirts to commemorate your efforts, you just get a lovely slice of cake and a well done from the fantastic volunteers, and that's enough. My third running of Charnwood was by far my slowest, by at least half an hour. I had been beaten by the most minor hill, a few hundred metres from the finish line.

Stories From the Field - Real Life Runners Saying Muddy Hell

Now I've done muddy races and marathons, but Richard shared a story that blew my mind: *'I ran a marathon involving multiple laps to make up the 26.2 miles. We ran through a pond on the first lap and each mile after that, so I had to cross it 27 times. Fortunately, I was near the front as it became very difficult to get back out of the water after a while. It was a proper pond, about five metres across, and the water was just above your knees in depth.*

Recently I was talking fondly of my memories of the Grizzly with a club mate Rob, and he agreed, *'The Grizzly Bog of Doom can't be beaten in the mud stakes, although the Dunstable Downs Cross Country was pretty bad a few years ago. The course was five miles of mud, and it was pretty difficult to run upright. I remember people slipping and sliding all over the place when we ran down a long lane with big tractor wheel ruts either side.'* That brought back a memory as I also did this race with Rob. It definitely was muddy and not a course for a PB that day. Thankfully, Rob, I and all our club mates avoided taking a muddy tumble. We both laughed, saying the mud is still on our trail shoes, and then John joined in the conversation too, *'Oh yeah, the muddiest race ever! I remember Dunstable Downs Cross Country. It was 2019, wasn't it? The entire course was a deep rutted mud track, and we were all a different colour at the finish. I remember that well. Going along a lane that was so slippery it was just about impossible to run.'*

During another chat with a group of my local running friends, they talked fondly of an event called the Welly Trail. Now you may be mistaken for thinking that you run in Wellington Boots, but the name derives from the club that organises the event, Wellingborough & District Athletics Club. In Northampton, a road runs from the town centre to Wellingborough and is known as the Welly Road. It's famous for a good pub crawl, but that's really going off-topic.

Vicki shouted out to a fellow runner Rob, *'Muddy races, Castle Ashby, The Welly Trail! That was the 14.5-mile half marathon, wasn't it Rob?*

Rob replied, laughing, *'Oh yeah, that's one of the harshest, just an extra mile or so. It was the gift that kept giving.'*

Chloe pitched in, *'The muddiest for me would be that Welly Run at Castle Ashby. It was miles of ploughed fields, and I took half the mud with me, even with trail shoes on. It was brutal. I remember clumps of mud stuck to the bottom of my shoes and I just couldn't shake them off.'*

Welly Trails and Dunstable Downs

So, the Welly Trail was to be my 70th half marathon. The mist settled just above the green fields on a cold February morning and conditions were excellent for running. The setting was the beautiful grounds of Castle Ashby, and their website describes it as *'The ancestral home of the 7th Marquess of Northampton. Wander through its gardens, which are open 365 days of the year, and you are taking a walk through history. Set in the heart of a 10,000-acre estate, the 35 acres of extensive gardens are a combination of several styles, including the romantic Italian Gardens, the unique Orangery and the impressive Arboretum.'*

As a kid, I went to a few country fairs with my mum and remembered buying delicious fudge from one of the many stalls on the lovely grounds. It was a wonderful setting to start this new local running event. With it being a few miles outside of Northampton, there were many local runners and friends from my running club. I was also a little nervous as I'd somehow managed to fall down the stairs the night before. I'd simply slipped on the top step, landed on my backside and my foot took out two of the banister rails. Ouch! I felt OK but was concerned that a bruise on my back or leg may hamper my run. The worry soon faded as I started strongly and walked along the road away from Castle Ashby House. It wasn't long before we ran into a field and through standing water from the recent rain. The puddles became bigger and bigger before we entered a ploughed field, and the mud was so heavy that it stuck to my shoes in clumps. After a few steps, it was like running with weights on your feet. I tried the tactic of stopping and shaking it off but soon realised there was as much mud clumped back on there after every few steps. I now had two choices, run or walk. I chose to run slowly, which was the general consensus of those around me. At the end of the footpath was a small gate with a friendly marshal holding it open and smiling at us hardcore runners who were already wincing at the toughness of the course less than two miles in.

Now you'd think that going from this thick mud to a nice flat road would be heaven, but it's not always the case. The road now felt extremely hard, and trail shoes don't always offer as much cushioning as road running shoes.

Add in the fact that your feet are wet from the last puddles and there's a hint of grit that's found its way into your socks, and it's certainly a challenge.

After a short loop around a village, we then had the delight of running across a path on the opposite side of the same field. Fortunately, this wasn't quite as sticky but tough on the legs, all the same. After completing a big loop, the following mental challenge is to pass the 10K point and see runners who chose this distance instead of the half marathon make their way across the finish line. I gritted my teeth and passed the finish arch, knowing I had another seven miles to go. Usually, this wouldn't be such a hardship for me in a half, but my legs were already screaming at me from the mud and wetness plus the hard surfaces. However, the next part of the course was a treat, going through woodland. I loved running beneath a canopy of trees, with wildlife and plant life all around. I saw rabbits and squirrels scurrying away from the pounding feet of us runners as we made our way over the firm ground that had mainly been protected from the rainfall.

After leaving the woods and crossing another field, we were treated to a short farm track that opened onto another ploughed field. This one offered a choice. You could either run on the sticky, heavy mud, just like the one before. Otherwise, you could choose the deep ruts that were full of water. Naturally, I tried both, and the first option seemed preferable of the two. The wetter option was too slippery and sucked your feet into the mud. After a few miles of slipping, sliding and shaking clumped mud from trail shoes came, guess what? More of the same, mud and then a footpath which was a little more stable underfoot.

I was relieved to take some respite and to try and keep my legs moving as my watch showed that I was approaching ten miles. To my right was a hedge with a gap and a fork in the path leading into another field. I suddenly stopped and couldn't decide whether to go straight on or turn right. In the distance, on the right-hand path, I could see some runners about half a mile in the away so I headed along that path. However, the two runners in red tops who I'd previously been following had disappeared. It was wonderful for a moment as the trail went downhill, and my legs enjoyed a break from the slog before. After half a mile, the path turned left and continued around the field. Suddenly, I saw some more runners coming towards me and some right in the middle of the ploughed field between us. Looking over my shoulder, some had begun running back up the path I'd just come along. It was very confusing. Two chaps hopped over a fence and said, '*Some idiot must have taken down the sign. It definitely isn't that way*' and gestured to continue the way I was going. I decided to follow them, and we ended up looping the field, back up the hill and joining the original path we'd left. Eventually, we saw a sign pointing us back on track, but there were a few disgruntled runners who'd added a couple of extra miles to their route. I just dug in and carried on. After another ploughed field, this time going uphill, I shook some more mud from my feet and then made my way back into the woods that I enjoyed earlier, knowing I was near the finish. Somehow, I got distracted and realised the fellow runner I'd been following wasn't in front of me, and the path didn't look familiar. Trying to trust my judgement, I knew if I carried on, I should join the path back into the field where the finish line was. The great news was that my sense of direction was spot on, and I was going the right way, but the bad news was that someone had built a great big stone wall some few hundred years ago and it now stood in my way. It was probably a couple of metres high and not climbable. I swore and then realised that I had to turn around and retrace my steps through the woods back onto the path where I'd last seen a runner. As I made my way through some dense bushes, a chap ran past and asked if I felt better. He thought I'd slipped off for a sneaky toilet stop behind a tree. I smiled and agreed to humour him before pushing my feet into the ground to start running again.

Finally, I saw the finish line in sight and dragged my legs through the finish arch to the claps of a handful of volunteers and organisers. I'd done a few steps short of fifteen miles after taking the two wrong turns, but I didn't really care too much now that I'd stopped running. My legs were caked with solid mud, much of which had dried and stuck to my calf muscles. As for my trail shoes, they would never be the same again. Even after two washing machine cycles, my socks from that day were still loaded with grit.

One runner complained that he'd run 16.5 miles and wasn't happy. He was comparing notes with someone who'd jumped over the fence at the bottom of the field where he'd pointed me back on track. They'd ended up going way off course. I chuckled to myself, remembering the vision of runners going off in four different directions and accepting that it was part of the experience. I guess I was never going to win this race or record a PB - it was just about getting around and enjoying the experience, which is what running is about most of the time.

The event was undoubtedly a favourite, and I ran it again the following year, doing the half again and entering the 10K in 2019. In 2018, the route was run in the opposite direction, and the ploughed fields were a little less sticky. Thankfully all the route markers were in place this time and I finished 15 minutes quicker.

At the time of writing this chapter, a club friend of mine, Zoe, shared a picture of The Summer Wolf Run she and a handful of others had completed at the weekend. She was neck-deep in mud, and it could've been mistaken for an army training video if she hadn't got a massive grin on her face. It certainly wasn't that muddy at the Welly Trail, but it was tough enough. As mentioned before, obstacle races haven't really been my thing, but I take my hat off to anyone who takes on the challenge, and Zoe is an absolute muddy obstacle legend.

Back on Track

Running-wise, I was back! I felt as if the mud was clearing following my collapsed lung episodes and that episode began to fall to the back of my mind. Over the year, I ran ten half marathons and recorded some pretty good times in the mid-1:30s.

Another local race organiser set up the Stanwick Lakes series, including a range of distances. The organisers were super-friendly too. In March, I did a time of 1:36:18, and June was 1:36:10, a difference of eight seconds on the same course. Ever heard the phrase, the camera never lies? Well, I can tell you it sometimes does. The race photographer captured a fabulous picture of me running at the front of a group in the first mile of the spring race, and it looked like I was the outright leader. Another small group had broken free from the pack and finished way ahead of me. I certainly love the fact that Stanwick Races use that picture to promote their events still to this day. Perhaps I should ask for image rights.

In the summer, I tried something completely different and had a go at a couple of track events. Kettering Town Harriers hosted two open nights, the first being a mile and the second 5,000 metres, or a 5K as I knew it.

Have you watched the athletics on the TV where each runner is called forward and introduced to the crowd? I loved this experience when doing the 5,000 metres, except there wasn't a TV crew or a crowd. When we crossed the finish line, runners' names were displayed on a giant scoreboard by the side of the track. For the Mile, it read Mark Kennedy 05:59:40. I was delighted to break six minutes and be only a couple of minutes slower than Roger Bannister in 1954.

The 5,000 metres was fourteen and a half laps of the track, and the temptation was to go more quickly compared to doing a 5K parkrun. I could smell a PB at the halfway stage but faded in the last few laps finishing in a pleasing time of 19:55, seeing my name in lights on the screen again. Not being a track runner, another unique thing I enjoyed was hearing the bell ringing to signify the start of the last lap. If you've seen the athletics on the TV or been to a race meeting, it's that moment when runners tend to kick on for that final push. I remember seeing many exciting races over the years: Cram and Ovett, Seb Coe, Zola Budd, Paula Radcliffe, Mo Farah and many others picked up their speed as the crowd roared them home. To hear that bell as I passed, albeit on a track in Kettering, was exhilarating. I didn't quite have the stamina to pick up my speed as the professionals would.

My running may have been back on track, but life was taking its ups and downs, just like the Charnwood Hills Fell Race profile. One minute, I'd feel like I was on top of the summit of a climb, but next, I was sticking and sliding in the mud, like that at the Welly Trail. Two steps forward and one back! Does that phrase ring true for you at times?

Jules was making a remarkable recovery from her treatment, and her hospital checks were returning phenomenal results, both fitness and health-wise. One evening, she came into the kitchen and started dancing, announcing, 'Jules is back!' I hadn't seen her dancing for so long and this made my heart sing!

We were building our business independently now and enjoying not having to work on someone else's terms. There were trips to schools around the country, and we'd built a great relationship with a funding organisation in Lincolnshire and locally in Northamptonshire. Aside from that, I'd been appointed a trainer for our network marketing business, which we ran alongside our personal development training company. However, fatigue and low mood were dominating my life. I'd finish a brilliant day in a school, get in the car, and Jules would drive us home. My brain would completely shut down, and I had no ability to communicate.

We ended the year how we began it though, travelling. After our magical trip to Malaysia and Thailand, we booked a month in Goa, where we encountered the amazing Goa Half Marathon amongst incredible food, beaches, people, sights and experiences. It felt like many of my anxieties would disappear when we left the UK. Perhaps we need to keep travelling. Hmm, now that sounds like an excellent plan.

———

Thoughts Running Through the Mind

Life has been likened to running into a headwind, and now the analogy of mud and hills can be added in too. We set the ship's sail in the headwind to keep us on course and arrive at our destination. Sometimes we need to ride the storm. The path can get sticky, and things can muddy our waters. Sometimes, it can be the influence of others or even something outside our control. Personally, I find mainstream media draining, so I choose to ignore it where possible. Even friends, family or colleagues can pass negative opinions and drag us back to a sticky way of thinking. Think about how you can stay on your feet and keep your balance if this happens.

I encountered many hills at Charnwood but got tripped up by the smallest one a few hundred metres form the finish. Sir Edmund Hillary climbed the biggest mountain on earth to achieve his goal of reaching the summit of Mount Everest. Runners complain about running up hills sometimes, but they're essential in our racing. An utterly flat run could be boring after a while. The best way to experience a view is to climb to the top of a hill and see it for yourself. Think about the hills and obstacles you may face and how you could conquer them to reap a big reward.

That small hill that tripped me up at Charnwood was more like a molehill though. Yep, the little things can make a big difference. Beware of those little pitfalls in life. Someone once asked me if I'd ever been bitten by an elephant, to which I replied that I hadn't. They then asked if I'd been bitten by a mosquito, and I immediately started feeling itchy. The little things do bite us from time to time. We could hear 99 positive comments and one negative, but the negative one will impact our confidence. Be mindful when being critical of someone else and be positive when being self-critical.

The small, seemingly insignificant choices in life generally add up to the biggest results. That dull training run in the rain, opting for a salad instead of a bag of crisps, switching off the news on the radio and listening to an upbeat podcast, smiling at a stranger or performing a small random act of kindness. These are all minor steps to creating positive habits. What habit could you create to help you climb your hill and enjoy the view?

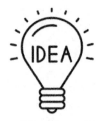

12. A Ton of Ideas

Do you notice that we humans love milestones, and 100 is a magical number? In cricket, it's a pinnacle to bat a century of runs. Footballers have been praised for being capped and playing for their country 100 times. A 100th birthday is celebrated by receiving a telegram from the Queen and now the King. The 100 metres is probably the most-watched race in the Olympics. Running a centurion, a hundred miles, is a significant achievement too.

My running mate, Sharky, achieved his goal of running 100 marathons and joined the prestigious UK 100 Marathon Club, which has hundreds of members. Many people think that running one marathon is a crazy feat of human endurance, so doing that many is just plain ridiculous. However, the local running community were in awe of Sharky's marathon journey, which is now approaching 200 marathons.

Membership of the 100 Marathon Club is quite strict. Firstly, and probably most obviously, you need to run an official event of a marathon distance. However, 26.2 miles is the minimum. A 35-mile ultra would also count, for example. Secondly, it must be run in your own name, and you must prove your finish time to the organisers. There are a few other rules, but it's an honour to reach the milestone and be officially recognised.

Sharky completed his milestone in July 2017 in Northampton, and a whole crowd of our running club gate-crashed the event to support him. After completing my morning parkrun, I headed down to the race to join him on the course.

The event was a timed multi-lap event. You get six hours to complete as many laps of the 3.3 mile course as you can, and eight laps equal a marathon. This was my first experience of one of these types of events, and I was pleasantly surprised, wrongly assuming that they'd be boring and soul-destroying. In fact, it was completely the opposite. It was as if everyone knew each other, and there were runners of all ages and abilities. Many were plodding around the course and using up the luxury of the time limit instead of battling for a PB. It's amazing how we can wrongly prejudge things without trying them first.

I felt a little guilty running on the relaxed course with Sharky and lots of our other members as we hadn't paid to enter the event, but it soon became clear that the organisers had embraced us turning up with open arms.

As Sharky approached the finish line, I ran ahead to get our members to form a guard of honour. A group of us formed an arch for him to run through as he took the final few race steps to the cheers of family and friends. It was a wonderful moment, seeing a friend achieve a goal, and the pride on his face will stay with me forever. After a short speech, we all shared some cake and went to a celebration party later that evening.

At the party, I chatted with Sharky and wondered if there was a 100 Half Marathon Club. I was now on 73 half marathons and getting close to the century, but I felt it would be lovely to be officially recognised. Here we go for the love of a target again. I found an American version, but Sharky came up to me a few weeks later, before a run, and told me he'd found it. The 100 Half Marathon Club! That was it; I was sold on the idea and had to look up what was involved.

The rules were similar to the 100 Marathon Club. The events had to be official, between 13.1 and 25 miles and had to be run in my own name. So, I set about the task of finding all my results and trying to verify the finish times, which was a bit of a mission as some of the websites no longer existed, and there were a few mistakes too. One event had me registered as Steve and another as Nikki. I did it though; after some painstaking work, I managed to get them all verified, and I was ready to countdown to the 100 milestone.

———

Real Life Stories from the Field - Sharky Bitten by the Bug

It wouldn't be right not to share Sharky's fantastic story here. So, here goes: *'My first marathon was the London Marathon in 2003, but I was naughty and ran in someone else's name (please don't tell anyone that, it's against the rules). I swore I'd never do another marathon but felt I needed to do one in my own name. After entering the ballot in 2005, I was lucky enough to get in legally this time.*

To help with my training, I joined a local running club called Rugby and Northampton to get support following a marathon training plan, as I wanted to beat my 2003 time of 4:45. My main memory of that day was watching a young man crying as he had left his running number on the coach, and it had driven off. If you have no number, you can't run. It was so sad to see. My actual run was uneventful though, but I loved the crowd and support, and finished in 4:35, so I was pretty pleased.

That was it! I thought my marathon days were done! However, a few years later, a work colleague inspired me to train again, and I entered three marathons in 2010. I decided to try different events and entered The Edinburgh Marathon,

The Wales Marathon in Tenby and The Snowdonia Marathon. At the Wales Marathon, a triathlete invited me into a group at about ten miles and instructed us all not to talk but listen to him, and to keep running. It was a very hilly course, and he dragged me around to a 4:01 finish. It was an absolutely unbelievable and incredibly proud moment. This prompted me to try for sub-four hours.

The following year, I got into London in 2011 and decided to change how I trained. All my runs of under four miles were run pretty much flat out, and among my running mates, these were known as 'sick runs' for obvious reasons. The poor colleagues who witnessed them didn't quite fully understand. All my runs over four miles were run at a solid 8:30 pace though, and the plan worked as I recorded three sub-four-hour marathons (London and Edinburgh in 3:52 and then Mablethorpe in 3:56). I was buzzing and loved my running. I then did the Dunstable Downs Trail Marathon and finished in the top 10 on a challenging self-navigation course.

Unfortunately, the buzz began to wear off when I signed up for a multi-lap timed event at Caldecotte Lake in Milton Keynes. It was freezing cold and there was a limited aid station. I finished in 4:13 and seriously started doubting myself. However, I ploughed on with training and entered the inaugural Milton Keynes marathon. On a wet and miserable day, I finished in 4:06 and decided that the training wasn't working after all. I pretty much stopped running, only going out very occasionally for a bit of head space. After eleven marathons, I decided to call it a day for six months and didn't run at all.

Luckily on New Year's Day 2013, my wife Tina and I decided to walk around a local reservoir. As we approached the causeway, we saw a group of runners clad in claret shirts, some pushing buggies, others with dogs. They were quite loud but clearly having great fun simply by going out for a run. I made my mind up that this was what I needed, to make running fun again. The group turned out to be Northampton Road Runners and, later that month, I went along to join them for a run and the rest was history. Instantly, I rediscovered my love for running and started entering events.

I didn't get into the London Marathon 2014 so I entered the Milton Keynes Marathon instead. A week before London, a different clubmate offered me their London place, and I took it. I ran a reasonable time but wanted to better it, so I decided to run a second marathon in a few weeks, and, surprise, surprise, I ran a bit quicker and was naturally delighted.

I then realised I'd run one in April and one in May, so I thought, why not try and do 12 marathons in 12 months? I actually completed 15 in 12 months.

During the Robin Hood Marathon, I ran with a guy, who told me he was aiming to join the UK 100 Marathon Club. I never dreamt I would aim to join the club too, but my addiction was well underway, and before I knew it, I was heading towards 35 marathons, then 50, then 60 and so on.

Plans were made to complete the magical number 100 in July 2017. This was an event called the 'Music Legends Prince Run'.

I've noticed there's sometimes a bit of respite as they do marathon number 99. This is known amongst runners as the 'flake marathon' (99, Flake...get it?), it's celebrated by handing out Cadbury Flakes to the runner and fellow participants.

On the morning of my 100th marathon, I was naturally nervous, but that soon eased as I saw fellow members of Northampton Road Runners and the 100 Club at the start. One lady had dressed up as the music legend, Prince, the theme of the run, of course. She had also bought me a good luck banner.

The format of this marathon was eight out and backs alongside the River Nene in Northampton. Many runners from my running club hadn't done this style of event but soon got to enjoy the friendly banter as we passed other participants. A bit cheekily, a lot of runners did a few laps without entering the event, but the race director didn't seem too fussed. My son joined me for the last lap, and as I headed toward the finish line, I spotted lots of clubmates forming an arch-style guard of honour, which was very emotional. Suddenly, I'd done it, 100 official marathons! Next came the presentation of my vest by a chap called Nick, who has now run over 350 marathons. My medal was presented to me by another runner called Paul, who's now run over 500 marathons. It's tradition to buy a cake and dish it out to fellow runners, which was duly done. A few beers followed, and in the evening, a surprise party was expertly arranged by my wife, Tina. Northampton Road Runners presented me with more gifts, and I did an interview with Radio Northampton. It was definitely one of the most memorable days of my life.

After reaching my monumental goal, I planned to not enter many marathons after 100 but not seeing people I'd met on the journey, I knew I couldn't stop, so what next? I decided to run ten marathons in ten days to really push myself.

The high points of my journey are the people I've met and the beautiful British countryside I've been lucky enough to run in. The low points are very few but usually involve not being able to run due to illness or injury. I think for most people who aim for 100 marathons, getting to the aforementioned 'nervous 90s' is just that. The thought of not being able to stick to your plan to complete on a specific date gets in your head and becomes obsessive. However, when you cross the line and earn membership in that club, all the bad races, illnesses and injuries go out of the window. I wear my blue and yellow 100 Marathon kit with pride.'

Sharky's story is inspirational. Obviously, knowing him well, I noticed that his running went from chasing times to simply enjoying the events as he then went on to push for the 100 milestone. I asked his thoughts on people who are nervous about running or being too slow. He soon dispelled the myth that having to take a walk break is a negative thing.

'It's quite common knowledge among my running friends that I have never run a marathon without at least one walk during the race. In fact, I used to purposely *build very short walks into my training plan. These days, I walk if I'm tired or out of breath but still try to hit the finish line with nothing left in the tank. I am a total advocate of running/walking. At the end of the day, you are still moving forward and putting the effort in. The main goal for me these days when running a marathon is to enjoy the occasion, the company of others and hopefully some beautiful scenery. Just keep on running.'*

Coming Out of Marathon Retirement

A few months after completing his remarkable milestone, Sharky picked a date and suggested that our club members run one of these timed events. I was tempted but had decided to retire from marathon running. Retired, listen to me sounding like a pro! Anyway, I declined politely. I didn't fancy going through marathon training again, and I was set on the 100 Half Marathon Club now.

However, on that beautiful backpacking trip to Goa, Jules and I were walking along a beach one day and chatting about some goals for the following year. Jules has always fancied walking a marathon and had been tempted to enter Beachy Head, a ridiculously hard event that some friends have done in the past. She asked me if I would walk the route with her if she entered. Naturally, I thought it was a good idea. I mean, have you ever been asked a question to do something you love doing and responded yes without even needing to think about it? I was in.

The conversation then led to, 'Well, if you fancy Beachy head, why not do the one that Sharky is organising with the club?' I was now talking Jules and myself into doing another marathon, and she agreed, so I was returning from marathon retirement.

It was an ideal event for both of us. The multi-laps meant we could see each other on the route if I fancied running, there would also be loads of support from my wonderful club friends, and the time limit had been extended from six to seven hours which meant Jules could walk the distance.

Upon returning from Goa, I sorted out a training plan which included a few half marathons. The first was my second running of the Welly Trail Half Marathon before taking on the Belvoir Challenge. The latter is a lovely off-road event in Leicestershire, one I'd done a few times before. It's muddy, across fields and farm tracks and finishes in a village hall. Yes, as you cross the finish line, you actually do run into the village hall. These events are extraordinary. There's no medal or goodie bag, you're just treated to some food and a delicious fruit crumble and custard. Ooh, and along the route are well-stocked cake stops. Yes, cake on the run and cake at the end! What's there not to love? This also helped me to tick off half marathon number 79, it was a win-win.

Effective marathon training includes a handful of 20-mile training runs, and this is tough to do on your own in the winter weather, so I teamed up with a few mates to increase my distance from the half marathon. These guys talked me into doing the Milton Keynes 20 mile. It was a long, two-lap route which I found tough and complained a lot to my training buddies, but it was an essential and sort of enjoyable exercise. I could also count my 20-mile events but chose not to as yet.

Never mind me though, what about Jules? I was totally in awe of her as she went out and walked for hours on end, sometimes in the snow and driving rain, building her distance up too.

Around 40 Northampton Road Runners made their way to Walton on Thames on an early April morning to take on the event which was called Leon The Runner. Leon was a runner doing his 100th marathon that day and the organisers, Phoenix Running, had dedicated the event to his name. We were gate-crashing his celebration and he was delighted. Race Director and founder of the UK 100 Marathon Club, Rik Vercoe made some presentations before the start to celebrate some members' achievements. One had done seven marathons in seven days, and another had done 52 in one year. Leon was cheered and wished well, and then he gave Northampton Road Runners a big friendly welcome and thanked us for attending. We then made our way to the Thames footpath to line up to the start.

The laps followed the path for just over a mile and a half before retracing the route. The first lap was jovial and fun as our club members joined groups and ran together. As we passed club mates, there was a wave and a cheer to each member, but these smiles turned into grimaces of pain and the occasional swear word as the laps mounted up.

Each time I passed Jules, she was power walking at a phenomenal speed and looking strong. I felt incredibly proud of her.

As we ticked off each lap, there was the reward of a visit to a table with the biggest pick-n-mix stand of sweets you could imagine. Like the Belvoir Challenge, what's there not to love?

The course was flat and easy on the legs, but there was one bridge over an inlet of the river, and we had to cross it twice on each lap. It will forever be known as 'that bloody bridge' or TBB for short. Near the bridge was a pub and the pub garden began to fill up with walkers and families who either cheered us runners on or looked at us in despair/awe* of what we were doing. *Delete as appropriate.

As I started my last lap, I was seriously feeling it in my legs. I'd really enjoyed running and walking with my club friends and encouraging those passing either way, but I knew I had to dig in for the final three and a half miles. There wasn't much time for stopping, smiling and cheering on this last lap and 'that bloody bridge' got sworn at twice more. I went past Jules as I made my way back for the final time.

Now, have you ever had a really good idea, that sounds like a really good idea until you realise it's not actually a good idea at all? Well, I had one of those in the final stretch. I picked up my pace and headed to the finish line. To end your race, you basically ring the bell, and your time is logged. My idea was to ask Rik, the organiser, very nicely if I could note my time but then try and walk the final lap with Jules. This would be a lovely experience to finish her first marathon with her and I'd also complete an official ultra-distance. So, I crossed the line to the cheers of the Northampton Road Runners crowd who'd already finished. Rik agreed to my plan and I went and announced my intention to my running buddies.

About 20 minutes later, Jules crossed the line to start her final lap and power walked past me. I walked quickly to catch her and tell her I'd be joining her. After 100 metres, I realised that my legs had cramped up far too much and promptly returned to officially ring the bell, much to the amusement of my friends and the volunteers. My time was recorded at 5:23:43, my slowest but most enjoyable marathon to date.

It was about to have the cherry placed on top of the cake though. After some chatting and story swapping plus some waiting, I saw Jules approaching the finish line and looking as strong as she did on the first lap. A ripple of applause turned into loud cheering as she got closer and closer. She looked over her shoulder to see what the fuss was about until she realised there a crowd Northampton Road Runners, marshals and spectators shouting to her for the last stretch. She crossed the line, rang the bell and after a big hug from me, there were hugs and cheers from the watching crowd. It was an extremely emotional moment.

Now, do you sometimes feel that someone else's achievement is more special than your own? That indeed summed up my day. Jules recorded a time of 6:47! To walk a marathon in less than seven hours is a remarkable feat. She'd also finished ahead of some runners. Our own marathon legend, Sharky, still raves about her achievement to this day. Likewise, I'm still proud of her too.

Hills, Hills and More Hills

Phoenix running captured me with the sheer friendliness and relaxed atmosphere at the Leon the Runner Marathon and it opened my mind to trying more of these timed events. However, I now had to uphold my end of the bargain and do the tougher Beachy Head Marathon in October

Life carried on its turbulent pathway with my brain injury and followed that all too familiar path of highs and lows. Anxiety and low mood were still dominating my weeks and I continued to try and press on. Running-wise, I did a summer mix of half marathons and 10K events, and the finish times were mostly good. I figured that if I carried on running, it would be good enough training to walk the Beachy Head Marathon course. That was to be a small error in judgement, as I was soon to find out.

We had some amazing highs in the months leading up to the marathon. As the summer was ending, we made a trip up to the Scottish Highlands to the Braemar Gathering. My stepson Russell had coached the army tug o' war team to the finals at the Highland Games for the second year in a row. We made our way up north to support him this time, and, in the preparation, he suggested that I enter the hill race. Like the upcoming Beachy Head Marathon, it didn't take much pushing, and I entered immediately.

The Highland Games were everything we expected. It was in a beautiful, old-fashioned arena set between a backdrop of mountains and hills. We arrived at the VIP entrance - yes, competitors got special entry privilege, and I was a competitor that day. We watched the games unfold in front of our eyes. Caber tossing, weight throwing, track running on a grass course and, of course, the tug o' war. Russell's team made great progress through the knockout stages, getting closer to the grand final.

The time arrived for the hill race, and I made my way to event HQ for the briefing. Just over 100 of us stood there looking either nervous or super-confident. The latter were the experienced fell runners who had clearly run up and down mountains for fun. The rest of us were first-timers and had no idea what to expect.

The race briefing was uncomplicated and went something like this, 'OK runners, you complete a lap of the arena before heading through this gate and across that field. You run up that hill to those five cairns at the top. Run around the cairns and then back down again. Don't worry; there's a smoke signal at the top of the hill, so you'll know what to aim for. There's no specific route so go whichever way you like. The only other rule is you have 45 minutes to enter the arena. If you don't make it back in time, we will have to close the gate and you'll be out of the race. Sorry, no exceptions. Enjoy the race! Oh, I forgot to say, don't worry, there will be a mountain rescue team on hand if you get into any bother!'

Mountain rescue team? What!!! The nervous runners looked even more worried now as the organiser stood with a sly grin. I've experienced many things in running but never a mountain rescue team. There was no time to think about that though, as we now had a few minutes before entering the arena. It was time to be excited as this was about to be an amazing experience. The gate was opened, and we made our way onto the grass track. The crowd of around 3,000 people made so much noise as we paraded our way to the start line for a good old-fashioned gun start.

The starter fired the pistol into the air, and we were off. A lap of the track with the cheering crowd was amazing, but I did my best to stay calm as we completed the loop and made our way across the said field towards the hill. Glancing up, I could see the smoke billowing out from the top and the cairns. I later learned that a cairn is a man-made pile of stones raised for a purpose, usually as a marker or as a burial mound.

As the hill became steeper, it became harder to run, so I reverted to walking and then climbing. It was like going up three stairs at a time in places. My quad muscles were burning by the time I reached the top, but I paused for a moment to look at the view. The arena was minuscule in the valley below. It certainly was an awe-inspiring sight. It was a climb of 1,253 feet, that's the height of the Empire State Building.

A quick check of my watch read 25 minutes. I now had 20 minutes to descend the mountain again. After rounding the cairns, I opened up my legs and began to let gravity do its work.

Suddenly, things became a little scary. Do you remember running down a hill as a kid and waving your arms like windmills as your legs would take you as fast as possible? Good! It wasn't just me that did that then. I was a guy in his mid-40s! This moment wasn't quite as fun as running down a gentle slope in my childhood days. I was totally out of control and had no way of stopping. My mind began racing! What would happen if I put my foot down a hole? OK, snap! Yep, got that! What would happen if I lost my balance? Tumbling and rolling! OK, got that! I had to find a way of slowing myself down. Throwing myself to the ground wasn't a good idea, so I tried to dig my heels into the soft heather beneath my feet. Thankfully my pace began to slow, and I managed to regain control, but I have to say, that was probably one of the scariest moments I've ever experienced in running. After reading Richard Askwith's book, Feet in the Clouds, I have since begun to understand that fell running isn't for the faint-hearted.

I had the pleasure of meeting Richard recently, and he told me stories of guys who glide up and down mountains and are so light-footed that their shoes barely touch the surface. I think I was a little more like Thumper this day instead of graceful Bambi.

My heart was racing as I reached the safety of a stone trail and decided to slow my pace. My legs felt like jelly, but I knew I still had plenty of time to make the cut-off in the arena. Fellow runners were sweeping past me, but I didn't care. I passed across a flatter muddy field and approached the gate, hearing the roars of the crowd. As I entered the track, I tried to slow down time to take in this special moment. It felt like the spectators were passionately cheering every runner home like heroes. I saw Jules, Roxanne (my daughter-in-law) and Warwick (my brother-in-law) in the crowd and gave them a quick wave before heading toward the finish line. The race officials shook my hand and congratulated me on completing the race. There were hugs and handshakes from fellow runners, and we stood and milked the moment for as long as we possibly could before being ushered out of the arena for the tight schedule to continue.

It took me just over 40 minutes to complete the race, but the time was totally irrelevant. I'd now ticked fell racing up a mountain off my running list.

Less than an hour later, Russell and his team won the gold medal in the tug-o-war final, and he was presented his prize by none other than the Queen. Braemar was unbelievable!

The following month, we had that magical trip to Majorca to do the Palma Half Marathon (number 82), and Jules did the 10K (as mentioned in the Run to the Beach chapter). After returning home, we were excited to be named finalists in the Northamptonshire SME Business Awards. The awards evening was on Thursday, two days before Beachy Head. Imagine our delight when the judges announced us as runners-up in the Business Innovation category. We made our way to the stage to collect a lovely, framed certificate. If that wasn't a big enough high, we were named the Best Enterprising Business in Northamptonshire a few minutes later. Yes, that's right, we won! We couldn't believe it! A business that the two of us had set up had now been named the best! We rose to new heights of imposter syndrome level immediately. So many fellow business owners congratulated us, and we felt like superstars.

Our smile was as wide as the Dartford crossing as we drove down to Eastbourne the following day. After collecting our race numbers, we checked into our hotel and went for a gentle walk and some food.

The thing about the Beachy Head Marathon is that very little of the course is flat. You either go up a hill or down one. There's a myth that people think it's easier to run down a hill than up one. This isn't the case; both can be equally difficult. I also subscribed to another myth that walking a marathon at a leisurely pace would be easier than running one. I was soon to be in for a big surprise. The race started on the promenade right at the end of Eastbourne before heading straight up a hill. The walkers began right at the back, so the path was muddy and quite congested by the time we were climbing. I remember getting to mile three in just over an hour and wondering if we could actually finish the event before the cut-off time of nine hours. Thankfully, the weather was good. It was cold, crisp but very clear, calm and dry, ideal really. We made our way up and down hills, through woodlands and around fields and managed to get into a good stride. It was beautiful as we began talking to fellow walkers. One guy told us he does it every year and has done it for the past 20 or so.

Time flew by, and we reached mile 20 at Birling Gap, a little inlet on the coast. There was 10K to go, along the cliffs past Beachy Head and over the Seven Sisters. It was almost at this point that someone decided to zap a touch more energy from our legs. The path was very uneven and slanted sideways, downwards towards the sea. It was extremely uncomfortable.

The Seven Sisters sometimes get called all sorts of unprintable names in this race, and they indeed were a test. Each 'sister' is a sharp climb and an equally sharp drop resembling a roller coaster. The surface is a mixture of grass and chalk. After over 22 miles of walking, our legs were now screaming. After finishing number seven, we learned that the route headed up a huge hill, just what we didn't need. We'd been going for almost seven hours at this point, and the evening was approaching, which brought a drop in temperature. The wind was biting as we reached the top of the hill, and we had around a mile to go. The sight of Eastbourne was welcoming. Navigating our way back to the big hill that we'd scrambled up earlier that morning, we just had to drop back down towards the promenade and cross the finish line. It was an absolute killer on the legs, but we did it, crossing the line in just short of eight hours. We were exhausted but delighted, and I announced that it was the most challenging event I'd ever done. That and Braemar were just energy-sapping in two very different ways.

One thing we were both very aware of was the fact there was a pub about 100 metres from the finish line. After collecting our medals, we headed in that direction and enjoyed the sweetest celebration drink ever. After ordering from the bar, a very kind lady pulled up two comfortable seats at a table and told us to sit down. We thanked her and accepted with delight.

Again, that day was a personal achievement in my 'marathon career', but I was so proud of Jules for looking really strong throughout. The following morning, she was bouncing around and so excited that we'd completed the Beachy Head Marathon. I was a little more tender on my feet. We'd beaten Beachy Head, but it had battered me a little more than it had Jules. My legs took weeks to recover fully, so I opted for parkruns and the local cross-country series until the end of the year when we went off travelling again. It was time for a rest.

———

Thoughts Running Through the Mind

This chapter evoked a couple of thoughts I want to pass on to you here. Firstly, I was so proud of Jules's achievements in running her marathons, and I certainly fed off Sharky's energy when he achieved his incredible 100 Marathon Club goal.

Have you ever been prouder of someone else's achievement than your own and used their success as an inspiration? We've talked, in other chapters, about self-comparison, but most people are keen to help others achieve their goals too. Who could you follow or maybe even connect with to help you on your journey?

Let's turn it around to selfless tasks and random acts of kindness and support. Since becoming an experienced runner, I've always enjoyed helping newer runners with their training plans, and one of my favourite roles at the local parkrun is pacing. There's nothing more satisfying than helping someone achieve a PB.

Who could you help on their journey by offering your experience and support? Who could you inspire to make some life changes, big or small? This positive action can inspire you to a goal too.

The second thought to consider is the goal itself! Have you set a goal with a measurable benchmark and then continued going and not quit once you've achieved it? Sharky and I have set goals to run 100 events, but we didn't intend to stop at 100. I have several friends who've set weight loss goals and used a target weight as the benchmark. Once they've hit that, they've carried on maintaining their fitness regime. Perhaps it could be a financial goal to save a certain amount of money or to reduce a debt by a certain amount each month. There are endless examples, but if you put a figure and a timeline on your goal, you have more chance of achieving it.

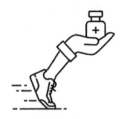

13. Randemic

Have you ever set a goal, been incredibly focused and then realised that no progress has been made? In the previous chapter, I'd set my goal to achieve the 100 half marathon milestone and then went almost a year without running one. My energy further diminished and focus was all over the place.

We travelled to southern India and Sri Lanka at the end of 2018 and had a wonderful time. However, I would have extreme panic attacks and felt anxious for no reason that I could find. Travelling was one of the most exciting things that Jules and I did. We loved it, but I was a bag of nerves.

India is an amazing country with beautiful sights and people, but it is also very over-stimulating on the senses, and brain injuries don't like too much stimulation at times. I managed to calm my anxiety when we reached Sri Lanka and had the most fantastic time there. The people are the humblest and the country is beautiful and out of this world. We spent Christmas Day on the beach, and I leant to surf. Well, I actually learnt how to fall off a surfboard multiple times. By the time we left this country and made our return home, I'd vowed to continue my quest for some counselling and support. Putting it bluntly, neither Jules nor I could keep dealing with this unpredictability that impacted our lives. As previously mentioned, I'd had some support sessions at the local Headway charity centre, but those finished once their funding ended. Other than that, I'd have my annual appointment with my neuro consultant at Northampton General Hospital's outpatient department. So, after returning from our trip, I made an appointment to go and see him again. He is a very kind and patient person who has always shown lots of empathy, and this time was no different. Instead of pretending that everything was sort of OK as I'd done in previous appointments, I poured my heart and emotion out this time. He offered to refer me for support at a local brain injury hospital. I was stunned! This hospital was less than 15 miles from home, and I never knew it existed. In fact, it was probably around the distance of a half marathon. I could've even run there. After being referred, I was given an appointment, and my life began to change for the better. Oh, and by the way, I didn't run there, we drove.

As with anything in life, progress takes a lot of time and effort, and this was no different. I had several one-to-one and group sessions, which was exactly what I needed to progress. It gave me a realisation and understanding of what anxiety, depression and low mood are and how to deal with the everyday effects of brain injury.

At the first group session, I announced to the group that I felt guilty being there. The other patients either had physical disabilities or couldn't work full time because of their brain injuries. I was the guy running half marathons and running an award-winning business while backpacking around the world. The old imposter syndrome kicked in big time.

No sooner had I finished my sentence when a patient's mother spoke up and said, '*You're here for a reason, and that is because you have a brain injury. Take all the support you can from everyone, and we'll help you on your journey!*'

I almost cried! For the first time, I accepted that I had a brain injury. It was time to stop fighting it and look at ways of dealing with it. As human beings, we spend far too much time trying to be something else or control the uncontrollable things in life. Some people live in the past and focus on the '*good old days*'. Especially as we age, we can slow down and lose the energy or focus that we once had. Instead of craving the past and the things that we used to be able to do, it would be better to channel our energy into what we can do. Brain injury had taken some things away from me and I'd spent years battling fatigue, pushing through, and trying to get my life back to what it was the day before my accident. I was tired though! Not tired as in I needed to sleep, tired of having no energy, tired of low mood, tired of anxious moments over seemingly insignificant things and tired of having little confidence and self-esteem. The biggest thing I was tired of was hiding behind a facade and pretending to the world that all was good. In all honesty, Jules is my world, and all the goals and things we love doing are in that too. Why should I be pretending to everyone that I was fine?

The year was tough, harsh and brutal, but it was the best recovery I would ever experience. In my time running, I've had regular sports massage therapy sessions; some have been painful and uncomfortable, especially after hard events. However, I know that the pain of this massage will last a few hours to a day, but the benefits would be huge. I now had to see my brain injury support as a similar process but over a longer period.

OK, you may be reading this and thinking, I don't have a brain injury, so this isn't entirely relevant to me. However, brain injury or not, we all go through traumas in life that could be helped or prevented by a positive self-care experience.

When I realised that travelling and running were becoming demanding tasks, I knew something had to change. Most of all, Jules and I live together, run a business together and share pretty much all the same life goals and values. I needed our world to return to the fun-loving harmony where every day was a joy.

There's a significant stigma attached to therapy and counselling. Firstly, many people feel there's something seriously wrong with them if they suggest attending a session. Thankfully, mental health is being more widely talked about openly now. Secondly, there's a historical hangover towards mental health issues, especially for men. We have phrases like 'man up' and 'boys don't cry', which can make it more difficult for men to reach out. Society has also placed a lot of pressure on the female population too. Women are also expected to be 'independent and display girl power'. Moreover, the media paints a high expectation of life. Social media feeds are flooded with the supposed perfect body, TV shows give an impression of the ideal world, and celebrities are put on a pedestal where we only see the best bits (this is until the mainstream media pulls them off their perch).

After a year in the hands of Isebrook Hospital in Northamptonshire, I was given tools, knowledge, and, most of all, support to help deal with brain injury. The pinnacle point for me is fatigue. The more I fight it, the more it becomes like a finger trap. Remember those things you'd put your finger in; the harder you pulled, the tighter it would get. If I fought the fatigue, it would affect my mood, memory, ability to speak, and concentration levels. Now I had these tools and knowledge. I needed to keep working on myself and putting them in place to help me move in the right direction.

After the India and Sri Lanka trip, I lacked the energy to run events. In one parkrun, I had a panic attack halfway around the course. I was running with a mate, and he'd noticed that I'd gone very quiet and slowed down, plus my breathing had become heavy. He put his arm around me at the end and asked how I was doing. Thankfully, he was one of the few people I'd opened up to at this point, so it was quite calming.

I ran parkruns and distances up to 10K but found it hard going. As the year passed, I decided I needed to enter a half marathon and get my 100 goal back on track. I picked the Dunstable Downs Challenge in early September, a few weeks before my favourite, the Northampton Half. Having done the Dunstable event before, I knew what to expect. It was an event with various distances, and the route was rural trails, hills and stunning views. On the day, the weather was spot on, not too windy, not too hot and clear enough to see for miles when running along the top of Dunstable Downs. I started the race at a conservative pace but got stronger and found myself passing quite a few fellow runners along the route. The last couple of miles retrace the path along the top of Dunstable Downs before heading down a hill and then a final mile to the finish. As I descended the hill, my feet felt like they were gliding on the trail below, and I had a huge smile. My pace increased along the footpath towards the finish before a short stint through a housing estate and back into the school playing field where the finish line was.

I stopped my watch, took a bottle of water from the marshal and immediately burst into tears. These were tears of joy this time. I felt elated! I ran straight to a big table full of cake and sweets, took some and picked up my bag from underneath it. After rummaging through the contents, I found my phone and immediately rang Jules. She answered, and I burst into tears again, telling her how strong I'd felt. We chatted for a few minutes before I headed back to the car for the short drive up the M1 and back home. I felt that my support and recovery were going in the right direction, but I was still far from where I wanted to be. However, like most things, small steps are the way forward.

It was now 2019, over seven years since my accident, life began to get smoother, and I felt my energy coming back. Yes, there were some dark and challenging moments. There were still tears, anxieties and panic attacks, but they lessened. I began to enjoy things I loved again. Running was fabulous, although I chose to slow down a little and not go hell-bent on times. Social situations became a little easier, and I felt a little more comfortable explaining to people that the environment was noisy, or I was struggling to remember points of a conversation. Travel was great as we planned an end-of-year trip to Asia again. We looked at Cambodia and Vietnam, but Jules suggested we go to Thailand because it was familiar. We had the most amazing trip, and I barely experienced a moment of anxiety. It was now becoming clear what all my triggers were, and they became easier to manage.

When we returned from Thailand, I had a bit of a blip, but I kept working with my neurologist on coping strategies and was determined to build myself and my confidence.

Half marathon number 85 was completed in Benidorm, and Jules and I had a fun few days there, as mentioned in the chapter, *Running to the Beach*. However, what happened next was the biggest spanner in the works as the modern world has ever seen.

A week after Benidorm, I'd entered a local trail run called the Peatling Challenge. It was a half marathon with the option of shortening the route to seven miles. My legs were quite heavy from Beni, and I'd agreed that I wouldn't push myself, so I opted for the shorter distance on the day.

Peatling Parva is a small village on the edge of Northamptonshire and Leicestershire. I'd made the short drive over in the morning and there was a cold March snap in the air. The ground was muddy underfoot and I knew it would be a challenging course ahead. After navigating my way over some muddy fields and along bridleways and footpaths, I turned a corner into a ploughed field and saw the darkest cloud ahead of me. Great, the route goes straight into that, I thought to myself. The cloud raced towards me, and the rain belted down from the heavens making the mud sticky. It was all good fun and part of the experience though. I really enjoyed the race and finished back at the village hall to be presented with a slice of cake. Now, am I selling running here? In fact, the medal at this event was a delicious cookie too.

Anyway, I had no time to hang around as we had a family dinner to celebrate my nan's birthday and I had to drive back and meet everyone.

As we sat down to dinner, the conversation was dominated by coronavirus, which had been spread over the media for the past few weeks. I rarely engage in mainstream news as I find it too shocking and depressing, but wherever you turned, someone seemed to be talking about this hyped-up story. After ten minutes of this chatter, I stood up and requested that we ban any further talk of this silly, scaremongering story that would pass when a new press story emerged. Two weeks later, the UK was in lockdown!

Jules and I watched a news clip online that showed Benidorm being patrolled by police cars, forcing people off the streets that we'd run around a few weeks earlier. We'd just hosted our book launch for *What The Hell Just Happened?* our story of brain injury, breast cancer and bereavement. Lockdown wasn't convenient! We had plans to speak at brain injury conferences and groups and help support families and individuals dealing with brain injury. We also had some exciting business plans and not to mention travel too. On top of this, I was 14 half marathons from my target.

Now, I'm not telling you anything new here, as we all went through the shock of the global pandemic and its effect on our lives. It brought us all challenges we never thought would exist.

As a committee member of our running club, we decided to cancel our weekly running sessions until things calmed down. The following week, I ran with three club mates, and we said goodbye at the end of the run, not knowing when we'd see each other again. It was surreal and terrifying.

The government soon announced that everyone could exercise for an hour a day, so that was it. I got to work creating some fun challenges for our running club members.

The first was based on the East Midlands Grand Prix Series, and members had to run and log a certain distance that week. Next was a virtual marathon challenge and then let's run a collaborative distance from Northampton in the UK to Northampton, Massachusetts in the USA. Once we reached that distance, we went to Northampton in Australia, passing specific locations worldwide. Someone suggested we continue until we'd run just short of 25,000 miles, the distance around the world. There were A to Z challenges, run every day in January and see how high you can climb by running up hills. We had a virtual team relay running against a handful of other clubs.

I absolutely loved collecting everyone's efforts and collating lots of random statistics. It offered us some sanity in a strange old time in the world.

Runners were then blessed with a rule that you could exercise with someone outside of your household bubble. My good mate Mark messaged me and suggested some fun challenges.

I co-host a fun local event called the Magic Mile, which we run at the local park monthly. Of course, this had since gone virtual as we could not meet up, and Mark suggested running it backwards. Unfortunately, brain injury affects my spatial awareness, so running backwards was out of the question. However, I offered to be the cameraman and film it. Mark did it and struggled to walk for a week. He then suggested another challenge called the Mark Run. We would run to local places that included the name Mark in them. It was great fun navigating our way from St Mark's Church to the Market Square and Denmark Road, among others.

The ideas got funnier and sillier! We had the Batman Run, Thomas the Tank Engine, The Cobblers Run (a local historic shoe factory tour) and the Immature Run, which was the pick of the bunch, finding locations with childish humorous titles. These included: The Rise, Norfolk Terrace, EsSEX Street, WEEdon Road, BUM Street (where someone had cleverly changed the letters from ELM Street), POOle Street, RockBOTTOM Discount Store, FarT Cotton and Butts Road. You can find the videos on YouTube if you look up MRMAK Running. The name MRMAK derives from our initials.

While on one of our fun runs, we also came up with the idea of the Northampton Monopoly challenge. In 2009, a Northampton version of the popular board game was published and members had to run to every location. It was great fun, and members posted their photographs on the route. Runners ran with fake Monopoly playing pieces from the dog to the top hat, and one of our members managed to get a police officer to pose as if he was arresting him for the Go To Jail square. It was indeed a credit to the togetherness and close-knit bond of the running community that helped many get through the difficult times caused by the restrictions.

Races Unlocked

You may have heard two phrases that both sum up how I felt at this point in time. The first was, *'that absence makes the heart grow fonder'*. Jules and I loved travelling, and I loved running events. Both had been cancelled and I started pining for them. The second was, *'If you love something, set it free; if it comes back, it's yours; if it doesn't, it never was.'*

Lockdown restrictions were eased over the summer of 2020, and we started to believe that the pandemic was on its way out (if only it were). Our running club managed to get back to meeting up in person again, and it was lovely to catch up with friends in small groups. Wasn't it comforting to start doing the things you loved again?

Jules and I also managed to squeeze in a week's holiday in Rhodes, and it was heavenly to be travelling again. The day after we returned home, I entered a local race called the Clipston Trail Half Marathon. This had been an event that was highly rated but always clashed with the Northampton Half Marathon. With Northampton being cancelled, it was an ideal opportunity to have a go at it, plus, it was equally heavenly to be racing again and getting back on track for my 100 Half Marathon Club goal.

Mark, the other half of MRMAK, gave me a lift to the Northamptonshire county border, and we excitedly made our way to the start line. Due to restrictions and safety rules, this was to be a race with a difference. Typically, everyone starts together at the start line waiting for the race official to signal to go. Due to social distancing, we couldn't do that. On this occasion, each runner was given a time slot to start. My wave was due to start at 10:20am, and Mark's was at 10:30am. The waves were then split into colours, red and blue. The reds had to make their way to one side of a field and the blues on the other. OK, I hope you're following me so far because there's more! Next, each wave contained 36 runners, and I made my way with the other reds to the said field. We were then all assigned numbers from one to six and told to stand by the relevant numbered post in the ground, but next to a cone, six groups of six runners were spaced out, two metres apart. Phew, this sounds harder than the race itself, but it was very straightforward and well organised. Finally, each numbered group was called forward and told to make their way to a table, one by one, and collect their timing chip before attaching it to their ankle and running across the start line. We were also required to wear face masks until we began running. The thought that crossed my mind was that the world was seriously in trouble if we were unsafe in the middle of a field with six other runners. However, the pandemic was serious, and the organisers did a fabulous job. Most of all, we were running back to doing what we loved.

I floated around the first few miles of the course, enjoying the farm trails and bridleways around the lush green countryside. I'd been treated to the beaches of Rhodes the week before, and now I was running a race.

The course was challenging, but I didn't care. It was just about getting around it and enjoying the experience. The course marshals were super-friendly and clearly enjoyed seeing runners back on their field. The last two miles were a testing uphill slog before navigating a ploughed field and then through a kissing gate. Stiles and kissing gates add an extra challenge to racing as they just break up your pace enough to throw your stride. At this kissing gate was another friendly marshal who had to insist that we sanitised our hands before opening it and passing through. The gate had so much gel on the top of it that it had run down the wooden slats and formed a big puddle on the earth below. Not only did my hands get sanitised, but so did my trail shoes. Passing through the gate, we had to hop a stile and cross another ploughed field into a strong headwind before a big downhill stretch to the finish line. I was elated as I finished half marathon number 86.

I did manage number 87 the following month, doing the Water of Life Half at Bisham Abbey. Sadly, more restrictions meant events were being cancelled again, and, before we knew it, the next lockdown arrived.

Like millions of other people, this had a negative effect on my mental health. However, I was determined to keep moving forward, step by step and get my anxiety, low mood and, most of all, debilitating fatigue into a controllable state. My group and one-to-one support had long since been moved online, but I enjoyed being around like-minded people. The biggest difference for me here was that we all shared the common theme of brain injury, and that wasn't a choice of ours. More and more supportive people came into our lives, either those suffering from brain injury or those living with a victim. This gave Jules and me much more understanding.

It was a long, hard winter which included a tough Christmas for everyone, but our family and friends stayed strong and offered each other as much support as possible. Mark and I continued our fun, slightly silly challenges to keep us sane. It was vital to have a good friendship and form a solid bond during such a difficult time. We'd run, chat rubbish, open up and pour our hearts out to each other and then laugh at some more fun ideas for the next challenge. Here's Mark's story.

—

Real Life Stories From the Field - Creative Running

'I guess I came up with the idea of fun challenges by just thinking about other ways to enjoy running. In lockdown, we were only initially allowed one period of exercise per day, so my mind started wandering as to what I could do in my local area. My inspiration came from things I'd seen online, where people ran marathons in their back gardens or around their area. I began by running 50 laps of a field which amounted to a half marathon, before going up and down a cycle path for another a week later. I would browse maps and come up with ideas to do to fill the time. Always enjoy trying to go off on a tangent and come up with new ways to enjoy the things we love.

When government restrictions began to ease, and we could exercise with one other person, running with Mark (the author) during those times was really inspiring. We got even more creative and came up with the Monopoly Challenge, which took our running club by storm. A simple chat ended up with something the whole club bought into in a big way. We came up with the name MRMAK by using our initials and began filming some of the fun challenges and putting them on YouTube just to make people smile. Feel free to look it up.

Dare I say that the funniest one was The Palinka Mile, just for the brutality of it and the fact that it progressed into an awesome day. We'd done the parkrun, followed by the Palinka Mile, then went into town to pick up our numbers for the Northampton Half Marathon the following day. We decided to have a few beers, which turned into a few beers more. It was a great day and the kind of day I absolutely love but not the best preparation for a half marathon. Anyway, you're probably wondering what the Palinka Mile was. It was four laps of a running track marked out at our local park. At the end of each lap, I had to drink a shot of a Hungarian alcoholic drink given to me by some Romanian friends, and it's super strong. Mark was filming me, and the look on his face in the video when he took a Palinka shot was absolutely priceless!

MRMAK and the challenges had such a positive effect on my life, as does my running in general. I've had a lot of personal issues to deal with daily which had a big, big impact on my mental health and anxiety levels. We all have coping mechanisms and ways that we use to 'escape' from these issues, running and cycling have been a big part of that for me. Joining my local running club back in the day was one of the best decisions I ever made. It's a perfect escape for me from the stresses in my life.

The idea of MRMAK came along at just the right moment, I think, for both of us. We were both dealing with the unprecedented times of the first lockdown and needed an outlet to channel some of the more positive elements of our life. It was out of these smouldering ashes that MRMAK was born. Two like-minded individuals deal with their issues in a positive light by combining their energies into something fun, positive and healthy, both physical and mentally. Please note that drinking Palinka while running isn't considered healthy though. Now the world may be slowly returning to a "new normal", but long may the MRMAK ethos live on!'

————

Thoughts Running Through the Mind

The pandemic was a tough time for everyone. It's probably fair to say that nobody saw it coming, and very few of us knew how to deal with the restrictions in our life.

There's a long-standing mythical debate that the Chinese word for crisis and opportunity are the same. One famous public use of this statement was during a speech delivered in 1959 by US President John F. Kennedy (no relation, by the way). He said, '*The Chinese use two brush strokes to write the word 'crisis.' One brush stroke stands for danger; the other for opportunity.*' In a more fun TV example, Homer Simpson quoted the same myth, saying that the word is actually '*cris-o-tunity*' Perhaps I'm going to show my intellect here and say that the Simpsons version reached out to me more. I use that word as part of my vocabulary.

Mark summed up a fantastic way of seizing an opportunity during the pandemic and went out to discover new routes in the local area that he had bypassed many times.

So, think about the time of crisis. What did you learn from the pandemic experience? Cast your mind back to the early days when we were confined to our homes. What did you do in those first weeks? Did you take up a new hobby or interest? Did you do something you hadn't done for years because suddenly you had more time available?

Personally, I noticed the calm and quiet around me because there was very little traffic on the roads. This made me crave more quiet moments in my life. I also rediscovered my love of art and began sketching historic local buildings, some of which have been sold in the town's museum. This wouldn't have happened without the gift of more time.

Did you make some changes and create new habits but have since let them slip away as life has returned '*to normal*'? A friend said he couldn't wait to return to work because his family drove him mad. I'm sure that was said in jest, of course. Another friend said they missed the commute to work. This prompted me to think of the opposite and ways to avoid being stuck in traffic or how could I better use my time if I was?

How could you turn negatives into positives? For example, the commuter friend could look at how they spend their time in traffic. Do they listen to the negative news on loop on the radio or listen to an educational podcast or something motivational and upbeat. Imagine a one-hour daily commute and listening to an audio teaching them a new language for example. That would give five hours a week of learning or 250+ hours a year. That would be more than enough to speak a conversational foreign language for sure.

We're all going to face adversities in life! Some will be minor and will pass quickly, but the same learning process could apply. What new, positive habits could you create daily?

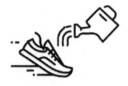

14. Springing Back Into Action

As the spring of 2021 approached, the world began to show signs of recovery and hope. Vaccinations were rolled out, businesses began to open, and family and friends began to meet again. I continued to remain optimistic, desperate to get back into a world we once knew, doing things we loved.

In April, I seized the moment to enter the Leicestershire Half Marathon at Prestwold Hall in Loughborough. A club mate Owen (the author of a fabulous book, Losing My Addiction), gave me a lift to the race, and we chatted like mates who hadn't seen each other for about a year or so. In truth, we hadn't! Arriving at the venue, there was a buzz as runners met up, chatted and smiled. The restrictions were looser than last year's event at Clipston. Social distancing was more of a suggestion, and waves of runners at the start were split into expected times where you could cross the line in pairs, so long as you were spaced apart. I felt strong throughout the course and kept a consistent pace, running with a big smile. It was glorious to have that energy back, the energy that had been missing for such a long time. My average pace was around seven and a half minute miles, something that I may have been slightly disappointed with in the past when pushing for PBs. Now, I'd realised I needed strength and enjoyment, not fatigue.

After the race, a handful of Northampton Road Runners sat in the spring sunshine and chatted, revelling in the glory of events being back. It was a lovely experience.

It was time to make plans for the run into the 100th half marathon, and I began scanning websites to see what events I could enter. An ideal scenario would be to do the milestone half at a local event like the Northampton Half, but that was only five months away, and to complete the remaining 12 would require a lot of planning and back-to-back events. It was doable, but many races hadn't returned to the calendar. I was also mindful of pushing myself too hard as well.

Number 89 was ticked off at the Olympic Challenge, a timed event in Northampton run by Saxons, Vikings & Normans, at the exact location where Sharky completed his 100th marathon. It wasn't until June when I managed number 90 at St Albans. On a sweltering summery day, I made my way around a challenging, hilly course and had to walk up a couple of the hilly bits late on. However, it was a fantastic event, and I was getting closer to the goal.

Realising that I was now only ten from the goal, I needed to make a serious plan. Mark and I (team MRMAK) sat down over a pint, trawled through more websites, and made some notes. He was as excited as I was and delighted to announce he had news of a free event I could run. Now I love the word free, so after a quick calendar check, I sent an email to the organiser of Enigma Events and secured my place for the Shaken Not Stirred Half Marathon in Milton Keynes. The event had been rearranged a few times, and numbers were down due to prior restrictions, so that's why free places were available.

After thanking the organiser profusely, I ran the two-and-a-half lap event at Caldecott Lake with Mark cycling around the course with me. It was probably one of the most humid days of the year and my shirt was soon stuck to my body. Mark lifted my spirits as I dug in for the final lap, probably a little less jovial than I'd been for the last stretch. His wit and humour got me around on a tough day, but he knew he had to do double the distance the following day as he was doing the marathon.

Running on a Work Day

Have you ever sat at work, wishing you had a day off to do something more fun? I used to have those days in the office, glancing out of the window at the sunshine and wishing I was on a beach, sitting in a pub garden or doing something other than being stuck behind a computer. I never used to imagine that I'd be running a half marathon around a forest though. These thoughts crossed my mind as I was on the first lap of the Salcey Summer Challenge hosted by Big Bear Events.

The sun shone through the trees casting magical beams of light across the forest floor. It was silent other than the footsteps of runners weaving their way through the trails between tree stumps and undergrowth. It was a Thursday morning at Salcey Forest in Northamptonshire, and, before setting up our own business, this would be a time when I'd be doing my 9-5 job. I loved the freedom of being my own boss and choosing to plan my work around my life and not the other way around. Running with others in this timed event was a joy. One guy was going for an ultra and looking to complete ten laps, amounting to about 33 miles. Another lady was doing another marathon. I forget her total, but she wore the coveted 100 Marathon Club t-shirt. I lapped a chap who told me that he weighed over 20 stone and was looking to see how far he could walk in six hours. Doing multiple laps and not worrying about a finish time was wonderful. It means you get to chat with different people who are all there for a reason.

I must mention that this event had an aid station at the end of each lap. Guess what was at the aid station? Yes, cake and sweets! What's not to love? Can you see the appeal of timed events here? No wonder I was doing my second timed event half marathon in less than a week. At the finish line, there was more cake to take home. Amazing! Number 92 was complete, and I had eight to go.

Running in the Park
The 24th of July 2021 was a magical day! It was the return of parkrun in the UK. This popular and free event had been cancelled since March the previous year, and thousands of runners and walkers had to go around 16 months without their Saturday morning fix.

I mentioned in a previous chapter that parkrun is the greatest thing ever invented in the whole wide world. Honestly, better than the wheel, sliced bread and even the internet. OK, that may be an exaggeration but I've been told a million times to stop exaggerating. All that aside, parkrun is one of my biggest loves in running, along with half marathons. Not only is it a free weekly event, but it also has one of the most amazing communities in the country, which is no exaggeration. Whether you can run a 5K in 15 minutes or walk it in 1:15, it doesn't matter. All ages and abilities are included, and various themes pop up from time to time. We've had milestones and anniversaries of particular events beginning. There's been superheroes events, Christmas fancy dress, we've had Olympians and celebrities visit our local event, and this happens at hundreds of other locations across the country, and the world, at nine o'clock on a Saturday morning.

Don't fancy running? Why not volunteer? There are several roles to fill each week in order to make these events happen. From marshalling to timing and briefing runners and walkers, scanning participants' barcodes to record their times, there's plenty to do.

My favourite role at parkrun is pacing. I'll stick on a bib with 25 minutes on the back and help runners around the course to hopefully achieve their target time. It's a win-win for me as I get to run, volunteer and help others, all in one hit. The great thing about it is you get to feel like a celebrity runner for a moment at the beginning. As the run director calls at the names of the pacers, everyone claps, and you can wave like an elite athlete does on the start line of a televised event. If you've no idea what I mean, watch the athletics on the telly and you'll see. I don't do that for personal gain, but it makes me smile.

I've mentioned my love of statistics, and parkrun is a running statto's heaven. Participants print off a personalised barcode before events, and it's scanned at the finish line, which logs the time. You can log on to their website and analyse your stats to your heart's content. Of course, you don't have to, but I love that part.

Here we go with stat time! As parkrun returned in July 2021, I'd been stuck on 284 events and had to wait a long time before my next milestone, 300, of course. There's a real celebration of milestones and parkrun award t-shirts for specific numbers like 50, 100 and 250, for example.

The return of my local parkrun was notable for another regular by the name of Bob. Now Bob was in his late eighties and had been stuck on 399 parkruns since the world locked down. It was an understatement to say it was emotional to see him finish number 400 after waiting almost 18 months.

Parallel Goals and More Saxons, Vikings & Normans

Suddenly, I had two goals running side by side: the 100th half marathon and the 300th parkrun. With eight half marathons to go, I went for another pint with Mark to do a bit more planning. There wasn't enough time to reach number 100 by the Northampton Half Marathon in September, so we began looking for other local events. By chance or fate, there was yet another timed event run by Saxons, Vikings & Normans at the exact location as Sharky's 100th marathon. This was mid-November and would be an ideal location to make a bit of a song and dance about it and invite some of my club mates to come along and join in.

The plan was to run two events in August, two in September, two in October and two in November. It was doable! Some would be back-to-back weekends, but I'd have a few weeks' rest between. I also wouldn't be racing them at my quickest pace, so it would be about running at a comfortable pace. A list was written out again and stuck in the front of my business planning folder.

Have you ever written out a plan and then fallen at the first hurdle? Well, I did precisely this. OK, it wasn't so much as falling at a hurdle but more about falling off a bike. My first August event was a Saxons, Vikings & Normans event, at, yeah... Sharky's 100th... you get the idea now. These were regular and friendly events in Northampton and usually ran over two days. Mark had entered the Saturday, and I was doing the Sunday. I agreed to return the favour of cycling around the course and supporting him, just as he had at Milton Keynes in July. I'd also chosen the Sunday so I could get my morning parkrun in first and work towards that 300. I drove the few short miles to the edge of town, hopped on Mark's bike and rode around the course to find him. He was about halfway around a lap and looking strong. We completed that lap; he took on some drink and headed off for the next one. I said I'd catch up with him and went to my bag to get out my phone and a gimbal to record some MRMAK footage. By the time I'd set up the camera equipment and attached it, somehow, to the handlebars of the bike, Mark had made good progress along the course. I cycled on a tarmac footpath along the riverside to catch up. One small section sloped up towards a pedestrian bridge to the left and then dropped back down the same level to continue straight on. I powered my legs on the pedals to go up the gentle slope and then freewheeled over the very short flat section before descending the other side. However, there was a slight blind spot by an overgrown bush, and I realised that a runner was coming toward me, so I turned to the right to give them space. The front wheel hit a groove in the path and flipped the bike sideways. I put my foot down to steady myself, but the bike flipped and threw me to the ground. In shock, I jumped to my feet before taking two steps and then sitting on the grassy bank. Two runners stopped to ask if I was OK, but I insisted they carry on. They were running a marathon, of course. I looked at my arm; blood was pouring out of my elbow, and my squeamishness took over when I saw what I believed to be bone. Another few runners stopped to check on my well-being as my complexion became very pale. Blood isn't my thing!

After steadying myself, I picked up my smashed phone and slightly scratched gimbal, uprighted Mark's bike and turned around to head back to the start/finish line. After washing my elbow in the toilet (well, the sink in the toilet, not the toilet itself) and patching up the cut, I noticed the giant golf ball sized swelling on my right knee, which surprisingly didn't hurt.

Mark finished his lap and came straight over to me, full of concern naturally. The first thing he asked was if I'd hit my head, which, thankfully, I hadn't. He then offered to pull out of the race to take me home, but I insisted he carried on with the marathon. He then continued to avoid his legs seizing up, and I said I'd call him later to update him.

The next task was to call Jules and tell her not to worry. She sighed as I told her what happened and asked me if I had been wearing a bike helmet, and I was totally ashamed to say that I wasn't. Honestly, I pledge that I will never ever go on a bike without a helmet again.

We made our way to A&E, and thankfully, after a quick x-ray, there were no broken bones. The next relief was that the nurse sealed the wound with some steri-strips, which meant no stitches were needed. The final bit of good news was my knee swelling was just fluid and should subside in a few weeks. The bad news, however, was that I wouldn't be able to run for a few weeks, so the August running plans would be out. There were a few bits of good news to follow though. Saxons, Vikings & Normans allowed me to defer my race entry until the November event, meaning I wasn't out of pocket. Mark's bike was badly damaged, but he got it repaired for free under a scheme for keyworkers from a local bike shop. Finally, with no races for August, Jules and I booked a couple of weeks in the Canary Islands. The indifferent news, I also had video footage of me falling off a bike. Thankfully, it didn't get into the wrong hands.

Back in the Saddle.

I'd lost a lot of confidence in cycling over the past few years, so taking a tumble on my first ride made me want to stay on my feet instead of balancing on two wheels.

After two frustrating and painful months, I did half marathons 93 and 94 at two local events, Cransley and Northampton, but I was behind schedule to complete the 100th in November. I was faced with a bit of a dilemma! No local events were planned in the winter, so that meant potentially delaying the milestone until after Christmas or doing an event that wasn't local. I toyed with number 100 in Lanzarote, where we planned to visit over Christmas. The alternative was to enter more events with less rest between. I had six to do in two months.

I'd entered two events in October, Silverstone Half and Rugby Half, both I'd run before. I did Silverstone with Mark, and we ran conservatively as he had an ultra planned three days later. After chatting around the famous Grand Prix Circuit, I wondered if I could get a place at the six-hour Rainbow Challenge at Salcey Forest. Big Bear Events had arranged this especially for key workers but due to restrictions, it had been cancelled a couple of times, and quite a few entrants were unable to run. The race director, replied to my email immediately that evening and said I could enter. Result! A beautiful course and lots of cake, remember? It was an opportunity for number 96. I ran a few laps with Mark, who went on to complete a 33-mile ultra.

How do you deal with knockbacks? Do you quit or look for alternatives? A few days later, I received an email informing me that the Rugby Half Marathon had been cancelled because of lack of uptake due to the restrictions hangover. I was out walking at the time and couldn't believe it. Another spanner in the works, as the saying goes. The organisers gave me the alternative of deferring my entry to the following year or swapping to another event. I remember that my mate Roger was running the Water of Life Half on the same day that Rugby was planned. A quick message was sent, *'Rog, are you still running Water of Life and, if yes, can I have a lift please mate?'* He replied immediately with *'Yes, and of course!'* After an email to the organisers, I got a surprisingly quick reply confirming my entry change, and we were back on track.

Despite falling over on a bridge, I loved the Water of Life event along the River Thames again. It was my third time running there and I now had three more to run.

I had another spanner in the works as no sooner had I finished number 97 before I received an email to inform me that the Saxons, Vikings & Normans beautifully named Chocothon had to be cancelled due to issues with the venue. Who thought planning to run 100 half marathons would be harder than actually running the events?

Out came the heavily edited plan with lots of crossed-out events and scribbles, and out came the laptop with the bookmarked websites to re-plan number 100. The plan was adjusted, and I entered the Baldock Beast, The Remembrance Run and the 100th was planned at St Neots, an event hugely popular with Northampton Road Runners. Oh, did I mention that Mark and I planned this over a pint? You can see a theme here!

By complete chance, I realised that I would also be running my 300th parkrun on the same weekend as my 100th half. What a double milestone that would be.

Real Life Stories from the Field – Running Blind

In this chapter, there has been a theme of improvisation and seizing the moment. At times, it's better to focus on what you can do as opposed to what you can't. Here's a story that really epitomises that.

It was around this time of my life that I met Darren who is a real testament to this ethos in life. A fellow runner had put out an appeal to help a blind runner complete a virtual marathon in less than four hours. That was a little too quick for me, so I reached out on our running club's social media page, and John offered to help.

Darren explained, '*I was so grateful to John for stepping in because my previous guide had to drop out due to injury. We had three months to train for the event, that was being run on the day of the actual London Marathon. After meeting up for the first time, we very quickly bonded and built trust. John faced a big task of guiding me on training routes to keep me safe. He did this by giving commands about potential hazards and making sure I didn't fall over or run into something.*

I was born with a condition called retinopathy of prematurity meaning I'm totally blind in my left eye and have very limited sight in the right. All I can see are silhouettes and shadows which makes it difficult to spot hazards when running.

I used to run on my own, following kerbs as markers to guide me but, my sight deteriorated over time and I realised I needed support. My gorgeous guide dog, Tilly, came into my life but I wouldn't expect her to come out with me on marathon training runs. She'd also struggle to shout commands as well. In all seriousness, a blind dog's job is to get a person from A to B so, she wouldn't be allowed to run with me. It would give the wrong message to her.

As we began our training for the marathon, I soon learned that John is longsighted and he joked that we were an accident waiting to happen. Of course, we weren't but there were a few tumbles and scrapes on the way. John would always feel guilty but all part of the journey.

I'd done a couple of marathons before, including London in 2007. I was overwhelmed by the whole experience and the day's atmosphere and will never forget the energy in the spectators lining the streets of London, encouraging all runners to keep going. I had so many mixed emotions: tearful, joyful, relief and suddenly the shock you've just crossed the finish line and received that all-important medal for which you've trained so hard. What an achievement. My first marathon time was four hours and two minutes!

Being partially sighted at big events comes with many challenges. At the 2017 Liverpool Marathon, I had to leave my guide at mile 17 as he couldn't keep up with my pace. Going it alone, I ran into a lady near the end. She stopped to talk to her family and bent down, of course, I couldn't see her and ran straight into her backside. It was slightly embarrassing but I managed to carry on to the end.

My goal was to break the four-hour barrier. The big day finally arrived. John had planned a fairly flat route around Northampton but arrived at the start with the news that he may not be able to run 26.2 miles. Only a few days before, his hip popped and he was in pain. I didn't know whether to laugh or cry. However, there were tears of emotion as several of John's fellow club runners turned up to help as a support crew. Loaded with painkillers and some supportive friends, we went off on our journey and achieved our goal, finishing in three hours and 53 minutes. I was overcome by the kindness and support of so many people wanting to help me.

This spurred me on to join the running club and become part of this amazing community. My story didn't end with running the sub-four-hour marathon, it's now given me a circle of friends in an environment that means the world to me.

A few short months later, I ran in the dark for the first time ever. It was scary because I can't even see the outline of the people in front of me and certainly have no idea of what was on the ground. However, I took the leap of faith and trusted my guide runner, whilst listening to their footsteps hitting the ground. I've also since tried off-road running which has the danger of planting my foot wrong and twisting my ankle but I love the challenge it presents.

Alongside John, lots of my newfound running friends have also stepped up to guide me around training routes.

'3-2-1… step up the kerb… pedestrian on the left and barrier on the right…' I need to concentrate on instructions like this which can be mentally tiring for me and my guide. It's also a challenge not to become distracted by conversation and chatter when you're constantly focusing on hazards.

This has given me a new lease of life though. Being able to run is complete freedom and a huge boost to my mental health. I'd be sitting at home depressed and frustrated if I couldn't run. My confidence is much higher now. If someone tells me that I can't do something, 'I'll say Oh yes I can', and start to look for ways how to accomplish it. Instead of thinking, I can't do that, I'll say, how can I do it?'

I'm eternally grateful to everyone at Northampton Road Runners and in the local running community who has made this possible for me. John is still like a mother hen, he sometimes lets me out of his sight but is like a parent who is caring for his offspring.'

Darren's story is extremely moving. Having a mindset to turn the 'I can't' into 'I can' is inspirational. Whilst talking to him, I thought it would be a good idea to ask John how he's enjoyed this journey. He added,

'I would never have seen myself taking on something like this. In fact, I used to describe myself as a bit of a loner and have never really been a people person. When I joined the running club, I was at a low point in my life but being around positive people helped me feel more positive. I don't know where I'd be without it.

When Darren's request appeared on social media, I found myself saying yes, why ever not? Running had given so much to me, I was ready now to give back.

Darren is an inspiration and he's given me the energy to take on new challenges of my own. I don't have kids but he describes me as a parent looking after a child and protecting it from danger. I feel guilty if he stumbles or bumps into things, but our inner trust and confidence have built over time and incidents are rare.

At a recent club night, Darren decided that he was going to jump some small hurdles that were at the end of each lap. I warned him that he'd probably face plant at the first one but secretly knew that he'd make it. Naturally, he did and it's heartening to see him trying new things with little fear. He has an amazing mindset to find a way to take on a challenge.'

Thoughts Running Through the Mind

Darren certainly has had a lot of obstacles to overcome to be the amazing runner that he is now. The key is how you react to a crisis when choosing to move forward or to stay still.

In the last chapter, we talked about the cris-o-tunites that can pop up from time to time. I certainly had enough spanners in the works when planning my run into the 100th half marathon; some of these were out of my control.

Humans can waste a lot of mental energy trying to control the uncontrollables. We use a quote in our workshops on creating growth mindsets that says, 'Effective people focus on the things they can control, and ineffective people focus on the things they can't control'.

Think about adjusting your goals when you hit obstacles that are out of your control. What could you do to get back on track? Another powerful quote I've heard from leaders is, *'Goals should be set in stone, but dates set in sand'*. This means that the goal is the focus, which should remain, but it's OK to make changes to the plans along the way and build in time if things don't go smoothly.

Avoid giving up because of a spanner in the works and ask yourself, how can I use that spanner? After all, a spanner is a tool and could be the best learning tool you could use. This is another analogy of learning from your mistakes and seeing them as growth points. There's a big misconception that failure is the opposite of success, because we all need to make mistakes to progress.

Make a note of some obstacles that you are currently facing or may have faced recently. Think about mistakes that you've made that could act as a learning point too.

Albert Einstein famously said, *'The definition of madness is doing the same things but expecting different results!'*

Think about what you could do differently to overcome those uncontrollable obstacles and errors in judgement.

15. The Flake Half and a Century

Autumn was upon us, and life was feeling pretty good. After much support from the fantastic staff of the brain injury team at Isebrook Hospital, I had tools and coping mechanisms were helping me to deal with the daily challenges that my hidden disability presented. Now I knew that fatigue was the main trigger. If I could become a master of it, then I could minimise all the other obstacles. Easy to say but not easy to do, of course! However, through a range of support mechanisms and self-discipline, like anything in life, it's about creating small positive habits one by one.

Firstly, and as mentioned, support is critical. Like-minded people who are on your side are so important. The only way I could get people on my side was, to be honest with them, which began by being honest with myself. I'd become more comfortable telling people about my brain injury and insisting that we move tables if meeting in a noisy environment or explaining that I was struggling to remember parts of a particular conversation. I found that 99% of people are really understanding and helpful. It's very rare that a person will hit back at you for being honest. I now have many wonderful friends who watch my back and generally notice if we're in an uncomfortable environment. It makes my heart sing when a mate or a family member suggests we take an alternative route because they recognise it'll be easier, not just for me but for us.

Another important step was to make as many things as simple as possible. I may have said before but I can become overwhelmed with lots of processes, like filling in complicated forms or taking on lots of information and even going through busy airport security can be taxing. Even if I've done these tasks repeatedly, the noise and overstimulation can quickly lead to fatigue. I've now embedded a rule into life: if something has more than three complicated steps, I ask if it needs to be done or who can help me with it.

One of the other significant tools is taking time out. If I need to switch off or even take a nap, I do it. Most importantly, I try to avoid beating myself up if the need arises. Anything negative will only lead to a low mood, which will loop back to fatigue.

OK, so I've just written lots about brain injury in a book about running and the positive impact on mental health, but these are all transferable tools. A good support network is key to anyone. If you're doing a Couch to 5K programme, then there will be others who can help. If you're experiencing stress that's having a negative impact on your mental health, good friends and family support is vital. Being honest with yourself and others will take a lot of stress away from life. If you're struggling with your pace while on a training run, your running buddies will wait for you. In life, an example of a big honesty you could display is the ability to say no. If you're unable to do something, be honest and say you can't do it.

The other two points are to make things simple and take time out for yourself. There's nothing more satisfying than some undemanding exercise like a run around the park, and that also doubles up for self-care as you're taking time out for yourself. Why do we make things complicated in life and rush around at a hundred miles an hour? Think about simplicity, calm and self-care. So, there you have it, transferable tools from brain injury coping mechanisms that can simply be used in running to promote positive mental health. It's certainly worked for me.

Beastly Weather

The rush of chasing the 100 half marathon goal also gave me a significant purpose. I shared the journey with many like-minded friends at my running club and the local running community. I'd even get stopped by strangers at parkrun who'd say, *'You're that guy who's doing all the half marathons, aren't you? How many are you on now? When is your 100th?'* These strangers would then become friends.

Mark also entered my 98th and 100th events and was ready to join me for the Baldock Beast. The day before, while making arrangements for him to pick me up, he asked if I'd seen the weather forecast. I'm not one to check the weather, but I discovered that gale-force winds and epic rain were predicted. Add that to the name Baldock Beast, and you have a huge challenge on your hands.

We drove south to Hertfordshire and found the small village of Baldock that hosts this annual event. Normally held in the spring, this one had been rearranged due to previous cancellations. We parked up on the edge of the village and looked to the right of the car, across some fields where the wind was blowing the rain sideways. Laughing nervously, we counted to three, opened the car doors and made our way to Race HQ to collect our numbers and timing chips. It was insane! We could just about stand up in the stormy conditions. We decided to make our way back to the car for shelter until the race was due to start. It was a good choice.

After half an hour or so of chatting, generally a lot of witty rubbish, we realised there were a couple of minutes until the race was due to start. I needed to go to the toilet, so we worked out that we could leave the car at 9:28am and make the official start time of 9:30am with the trip to the portaloo. The countdown was repeated, and we opened the car doors and made our way to the start line via the toilet. I'm sure this is probably too much information here, but the male portaloos at some events are stand-up urinals. I visited this pop-up convenience for a pre-race relief and then realised the meaning of the well-used phrase 'peeing in the wind.' You must have heard it before, I'm sure?

I found Mark sheltering behind a portaloo, and I suggested we return to the car and get our rain jackets and beanie hats. At least they'd provide some relief against the elements.

Now, most people would stay in the car or even drive home and give up, but there was some kind of sadistic fun in the challenge that lay ahead. When you love running, I guess this is the sort of thing you do.

The first few miles of the route ran out along a combination of country lanes and trails. The rain was lashing across the fields at a 90-degree angle and hitting our right-hand side with some real force. We both had our hats on sideways and could barely hear each other in conversation. A river-like stream of water ran down the side of the road. Sometimes, it was impossible not to run through. We got some respite from the wind when running alongside hedges next to the road. One thing is for sure, the whole field of runners was in it together, and everyone supported each other. There was plenty of humour blowing around in the wind.

If it was tough on the runners, it was even tougher on the marshals, who had been standing at various points on the course, battling to stay upright but still managing to hand out water and cheer everyone on.

Halfway into the route, we were treated to a lap of a beautiful village before heading through a woodland trail, which was muddy and wet. It was totally enjoyable all the same. After ten miles of wind and rain, the weather began to subside, and the sky brightened. A mile later and the sun broke through, and by the time we were running along the finish stretch, you wouldn't have known there had been a storm except for a few puddles at the side of the road.

Despite not loving running in the wind, I really enjoyed this event and the camaraderie that it brought between everyone involved. It was a beast of a morning but one that gave us some good memories. I was now on the home straight and only had to cover a marathon distance of 26.2 miles in total. I had a couple of weeks' rest before back-to-back events.

The Flake Half

Did I hear someone mention cake? I keep trying to sell this running lark with the reward of cake, don't I? Well, half marathon 99 guaranteed just that.

I'd entered the Remembrance Run organised by Zig Zag Running, another master of timed events. It took place on Remembrance Sunday at Hinchingbrooke Country Park in Cambridgeshire

When entering, there was a box in the online form asking if you had any special milestones to celebrate at the event. Of course, these events are common ground for the 100 Marathon Club members and those working towards it. I wrote in the box that it was my 99th half marathon.

The day before, as I was checking my travel arrangements and making sure I was aware of the day's instructions, I noticed some delicious cakes on the Zig Zag Events Facebook page. The caption accompanied one photograph, 'Here's Mark's Flake Half Cake!' It suddenly dawned on me that this was to commemorate my 99th half. Flake = 99, of course. How special did I feel? It was an amazing gesture.

Upon arrival, I collected my race number, which was, yep, number 99. The race briefing included several milestone announcements in which my 'Flake Half' was celebrated. Runners were also informed that there would be a two-minute silence at eleven o clock for Remembrance Day. A whistle would sound, and wherever you were on the course, you would stop to observe it.

The race started, and the route immediately followed a forest trail up a hill before turning into a denser wooded path. I was smiling and had goosebumps on my arms as I ran through the sheer beauty, passing a few runners and meeting walkers in the opposite direction. The first marshal called out my name and cheered on my 99th half. Every single marshal repeated this throughout the course; they were all aware of everyone's special races today. It was really touching. After leaving the woodland, I had four laps of this beautiful course that followed a very muddy trail and then looped around a reservoir before another woodland route. It was heaven!

After each lap, there was the customary cake and sweet stand, plus a chance to hydrate too. Oh, how I love these events. After crossing the line in a pretty reasonable time, I made my way to the country park's community centre to sample a slice of my Flake cake. Everyone was so friendly and genuinely enjoyed welcoming runners to the event. A lovely lady behind the cake table loaded me up with a couple more slices to take away, and I vowed that I'd return soon to participate in another one of their races.

As I made my way outside, the whistle sounded for the two-minute silence, and the whole area fell beautifully peaceful, other than the faint noise of wildlife in the distance.

Ton Up

The following Saturday, I walked across the road to my local park and met some Northampton Road Runners and parkrun friends to celebrate my 300th parkrun. It was also my 250th at the Northampton venue, so a double milestone, I guess. Starting right at the very back, I made my way through the field, chatting to friends along the way. This is a great tactic to avoid pushing too hard, and it's also very sociable. At the finish line, there was some cheering from a few friends before a few photographs and sharing some chocolates I'd brought along. It was a beautiful November morning with ideal conditions to mark milestone number one of the weekend.

The following morning, Mark arrived excitedly to pick Jules and me up for the short trip to St Neots in Cambridgeshire. We drove there, full of chatter. I'd arranged a meeting point at a pub near the finish line so we could meet for a milestone pint afterwards. Around 40 members from our club were running the event so that it would be pretty special.

I planned to run around the course with Mark and simply enjoy the race. Now, you know how something simple could go so wrong in a few moments? I'd headed inside to the bag drop to leave my change of clothes in the storage area as Mark made his way to the portaloos outside. Spotting an inside toilet, away from the cooler outdoors, I decided to seize the opportunity for some pre-race relief. I underestimated how long the queue was, but I was now committed and decided to wait. Thankfully, I found Jules outside, who walked with me to the start line and gave me a pre-race hug and a good luck kiss. I heard the countdown to the start. We had a minute to go. Wandering through the crowded field, I chatted to a few fellow club members who were excited about my run. I felt a little nervous for some reason. Someone then told me that Mark was up ahead.

The race started, and I settled into a good early pace, passing a few mates in their club colours and chatting to them. Then I saw Mark a few hundred metres in front and thought I could catch him in a few minutes. I knew a nice downhill stretch was coming up where I could open up my legs in the second mile. As I closed in on Mark, I spotted one vital flaw - it wasn't him. It was a fellow club runner who was running at a solid pace. This was three miles in and I was feeling really strong, so the obvious thing was to keep going at the same pace. A couple of miles later, I passed the pacer with one hour and 45 minutes on his back, and, at the halfway point, I was on target for breaking one hour 40 minutes. Suddenly the enjoyable plod became thoughts of aiming for my quickest half marathon for over four years. It would be nowhere near a PB, but it would be a good milestone in my recovery from a few years of mental anguish.

The final miles of the route go from flat to a nice downhill one-mile stretch back into St Neots. As I reached the crest of the hill, I looked at my watch and guessed a time of 1:38 before planning my finish line celebration to salute the 100th half marathon. My mind was racing with excitement.

'Ooh, my legs feel great. A quick check of the watch, three-quarters of a mile to go, and the pace is good. I'm going to catch that guy in front. Yay caught him, but this isn't a race remember. Woohoo, over a humpback bridge, but be careful; you don't want to fall now. That would be a disaster. Oh no, what happens if I fall? OK, stop thinking about that. Think about punching the air repeatedly as you cross the line. Yeah, I'm going to punch the air as soon as I see Jules and my running mates. What a moment that would be. I'll see that corner where we turn left to the finish any minute now. There it is, I can see it, nearly there now. I can hear the crowd. Remember the fist-pumping in the air. Here's the corner; around we go. Yesssss, I can see the finish line. OK, look cool, don't sprint, just keep the pace going. Only a few more steps until I start the fist-pumping. There are some Northampton Road Runners; give them a wave. Yesssss waved and first fist-pump into the air. Yeahhhhhh, there's Jules, woohoo. Both arms are waving in the air now, and here come the tears of emotion. Please go on, race announcer, call out my name. Go on... 'Number 689, Mark Kennedy,... yes, he called out my name.'

I crossed the line and felt ecstatic. Looking around, fellow runners could've easily mistaken this moment of delight as celebrating my first half marathon, not my 100th. Honestly, the emotion was like that September day some 14 years earlier.

Jules came running over and gave me a big hug, despite my sweaty running shirt. She was so proud. Next, a couple of club mates headed in my direction to offer handshakes and hugs. I grabbed a drink and was presented with my finisher medal by a friendly volunteer before telling him it was my 100th half marathon. He congratulated me before handing the next medal to the next finisher behind me.

Moments later, an arm wrapped around my shoulder, and it was Mark. '*Congratulations buddy, I got stuck in the toilet at the start!*' I laughed when he told me that he missed the whole race start due to a pre-run visit to the portaloo taking a little longer than he'd anticipated. Anyway, at the risk of too much information, we then headed back to the crowd of Northampton Road Runners to cheer on the remainder of the field. There were more handshakes and congratulatory hugs from friends.

As the rest of our runners came home, we headed to the pub for a lovely rest on the sofa and celebrated with a pint or two.

A messed-up race plan ended up being my fastest half for four years with a time of 1:38:22; that's exactly seven and a half minute miles. This would've been a time I would've been slightly disappointed with when chasing PBs, but now I was elated. Most importantly, I'd reached the 100 half marathon goal and joined an exclusive club of fellow runners who'd logged their efforts and submitted them to the organisers. The next simple task the following day was to email my spreadsheet over with one extra line added in reading number one hundred. A few weeks later, my 100 Half Marathon t-shirt arrived in the post which I now wear with pride.

―――

Real Life Stories from the Field – Runners Encouraging Others

In the Randemic chapter, Mark, the other half of MRMAK, told his story of maintaining sanity during a crisis and the positive effect running has on his mental health. I've decided to bring him back here to talk more about some of the above memories, supporting me and to mention his running goals.

'Being a part of Mark's journey and encouraging him to get to the 100th half marathon was very satisfying and a whole lot of fun.

We did the Baldock Beast event on a wet Sunday morning, and I just remember horizontal rain when I opened the car door that managed to get Mark drenched while he was still sitting in the passenger seat! It probably would've been best starting that run in a wetsuit with flippers. It was bonkers! However, running together and supporting each other made us want to get out of the car and actually run the race. It would've been much less fun running it solo.

After making the final plans for the 100th half marathon at St Neots Half, I simply had to be there to share the moment with Mark and a whole load of members from our brilliant running club. It was a late start for me, 'delayed' by a toilet visit. I came out of the loo, and nobody was around. The race had started about ten minutes earlier, and it took me just over a mile to catch the tail walkers at the back of the field. I spent the rest of the run picking my way through the field, and it turned out to be a very social event as I've never had the chance to talk to so many fellow club runners during a race. Although they all said the same thing, 'Ooh, Mark was looking for you at the start.' MRMAK were finally reunited at the finishing line to start the 100th half celebrations.

As you can tell, I love my running and am always looking for the next rush of a fun challenge. It would be nice to get to 100 marathons and 100 half marathons, ideally at the same time, which would be pretty epic. It's also gratifying to help friends get into running and introduce people into my running club who have gone on to such great things. I was proud to see them winning awards and achieving so much with their running. Also, helping friends around their first race event or to achieve a PB gives me an enormous sense of satisfaction.'

Thoughts Running Through the Mind - What Next?

Have you reached a milestone and wondered what to do next? How did you feel? Sometimes it's normal to feel the post-event blues. For example, I have friends who experience a real comedown after completing their first marathon. They'd trained hard for months on end, had the buzz of the day, crossed the finish line, and then, suddenly, what next?

I call this a '*danger point!*' There's a danger of quitting and giving up. There's also a danger that you'll enter another marathon, of course, and become addicted. Joking aside though, this can be a critical point for an individual in moving to the next step on their goal list. So, think about a time when you've achieved something significant, and perhaps it's something that you'd like to pick up again. Maybe you're still doing something, but you could renew your vows and appreciate your love of whatever it is.

I'm lucky enough to live close to a beautiful park (home of the Northampton parkrun, of course). I've been guilty of getting tired of walking or running around the same park over the past so many years. However, it became my go-to sanctuary when restrictions were placed on us. I noticed little beauties in the park that I'd forgotten or taken for granted. It became my mission to visit it daily during lockdowns and explore it repeatedly.

Likewise, my half marathon journey continues, and I'm constantly looking at new events and old favourites to enter. Writing this book has reminded me of some lovely places I need to revisit.

The MRMAK stories sound like a couple of mates having a bit of fun, but the serious point is that we discovered some new challenges we hadn't thought of before. Mark helped me around some events on my journey to the 100, but I've done the same for him. This included turning up unannounced to the start of my 101st half marathon while he was about to start the marathon. We ran the first half together. This is something I see a lot in running, where people help and support each other.

If you have a goal that you've not yet achieved, keep planning and working towards that goal but think about your plan after achieving it. The most straightforward question to ask yourself is, '*What next?*'

The second question is, '*Who's that person who can help and support you along the way?*' Find your cheerleader and work towards like-minded goals.

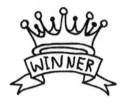

16. Winner, Winner, Veggie Dinner

The 100 Half Marathon Club was a goal of mine, and it felt like a victory. Running is all about personal challenges and being your best. It doesn't matter if you come first or somewhere near the back of the field, this book has shown all levels and abilities are welcome in this sport. That also applies to life. Some people will be better, but you don't need to be at the top of the pile to be your best. However, I've been fortunate enough to finish in first place at some events and feel a little glory.

Also, a few years ago, I switched to a plant-based diet purely for health reasons. That's why I decided to call the chapter Winner, Winner, Veggie Dinner. I've heard the phrase Winner, Winner, Chicken Dinner many times, and chicken is an excellent source of protein which is essential to form part of a diet required for running, but I decided to use the phrase veggie dinner for a bit of fun.

When I began running, I had little idea of nutrition or how to fuel myself for races. There was lots of talk about carb loading, which usually involved eating loads of pasta. When I discovered the love of running, I became fascinated with nutrition and enrolled on a course, even briefly running a sports nutrition business. Although I took a different route away from maintaining the core of my business, it was good to learn a lot about the functioning of our bodies.

Winning Races
I've talked about finishing first in the Parklands Jog and Run one-mile fun runs, but I wondered what it would be like to cross the line first in some other distances. In 2019, I had that experience returning to the Kettering Harriers Open Track Night. On entering the event, you had to list your expected time, and then you'd take part in the run based on that assumption. I was running 5K in around 21-22 minutes at the point, so I entered the 20-25 minute wave. Competitors were treated with our names being called out as we stepped forward to the start line. Like the previous track events I'd done there before, the starter fired a pistol, and the race was away. It was a

calm and cool night for July, with ideal conditions. I settled into a good pace and began to pull away from the rest of the field. Five kilometres is fourteen and a half laps of a running track, so it's quite a lot of loops. I'd lapped the entire field with two laps to go and felt invincible. The bell sounded for the final lap, and it was exhilarating to be the first runner with 400 metres to go. I crossed the line in 20:59 and felt absolutely delighted.

Now, I must add, this wasn't a competitive event with no medal or award at the end, but I thought, I'm going to take this as a first-place finish.

When watching the sub-20-minute race being run after ours, I was pleased that I'd entered my chosen wave. I would've finished second last in the elite race.

In the chapter Springing Back to Action, I mentioned the Saxons, Vikings & Normans Olympic Challenge, a timed event. This was half marathon number 89, but it was also quite special as I was the first to finish the half distance on this day. Runners were set off in waves due to the restrictions still being in place. When I crossed the line and checked my finish time, the organisers presented me with a medal and stuck a badge on it with 'First Finisher'. I knew I had to take that as my first place in a half marathon.

Now, as I'm telling you these stories of finishing first, I'm writing this with a lot of imposter syndrome. The Olympic Challenge first-place finish was 15 minutes slower than my PB and is also way slower than the winner of many of the half marathons I've run. However, that doesn't matter, it's on my running CV, and I'm happy to be proud of my achievements.

First Across the Line

After completing my 100th half marathon, I had two choices. Stop running them or enter another. I did the latter and raced only a few weeks later, returning to Hinchingbrooke Country Park where I did my 'Flake Half'. It was a lovely wintery run through the woods and my last race of the year for number 101. My goal then became about enjoying half marathons and keeping running the distance, so I planned a few more for 2022, including the Saxons, Vikings & Normans in Northampton. Remember, I'd missed the first one due to falling off a bike the day before and then the following date was cancelled in my run into the 100?

After a quick email to the organiser Traviss, I was booked in for the next date in Northampton, which was set for the Easter weekend. I chose the Sunday, which was named the Chocothon. Yes, that's right, chocolate at a run. I've mentioned cake loads but I love chocolate more.

Have you ever planned something and then realised you've dropped a clanger? No sooner had the email arrived in my inbox confirming my entry did I realised we had family coming on Sunday, so I hit reply and asked to change to Saturday instead. The bad news was, it wasn't called the Chocothon on Saturday, but the good news is, it was the Cakeathon. Yes, cake at a run – oh well!

A week before the race, it was the monthly running of the Magic Mile, an event that I helped host at our local park after parkrun. I love this event because we have a small cult following of around 20 or so runners who try to enter every time. Then, a handful of parkrunners stay on and run, jog, walk or even wheelchair around the mile loop. It's a straightforward, no-frills event where we record everyone's time, and they can measure their runs over quite a unique distance. The original organiser had the course officially measured when he first set it up, so we could even count it as an official event if we wanted to.

Usually, I announce the event and time it, but we had a few extra volunteers on this occasion, so they suggested I run it that day. I'd done parkrun and hadn't felt particularly energetic and debated last minute about passing up the opportunity but decided to go for it. It would also be a good chance to have a race with my mate Mick and reignite our fun battles of old. As we made our way to the start, a couple of speedy runners, who usually do the mile, came over and apologised that they couldn't do it today. One had an appointment, and the other had a niggling injury. Mick and I then chatted on the short walk to the start line about the potential of winning the Magic Mile. I got into an early lead on Mick and then waited as he has a habit of finding a second wind generally in the second half of the race. The rush didn't come, and I crossed the line in first place.

Warning, imposter syndrome time! The big hitters weren't there, it was a race I organised, the field was small, and it was nowhere near my fastest mile. Yep, all the excuses came out as I shook Mick's hand at the end. However, I added a first-place finish in a mile to my glittering running career.

Chocs Away

A week after the Magic Mile glory, I was at the start line for the Cakeathon. It was the fourth attempt to get here, but I'd made it and was ready to run.

There was a lovely welcome from the organiser and owner of SVN, Traviss. He and the volunteers had remembered my bike crash and asked how I was. I showed them my battle scars before we had a short race briefing. Travisss explained the route of the 5.3 miles lap that would be repeated as often as required to complete your desired distance. He then said, '*If you don't know where you're going, follow Mark, he's local!*' I just happened to be standing at the front, so I smiled and set up my watch before we were counted down for the start.

The start/finish is at a hotel car park, and the route then crosses a bridge before heading alongside the River Nene (pronounced Nenn if you're from Northampton and Neen by anyone else). You then follow this cycle path, past the very deep groove in the tarmac, big enough to dislodge a rider from their bike, it then turns onto a mixed grassy stony track that crosses a bridge and loops around a huge reservoir-type lake. After the loop, you retrace your steps back to the hotel and record your lap.

I turned onto the cycle path and eventually passed that hazardous spot where I'd taken my tumble. After a mile, I realised that I couldn't hear the footsteps or heavy breathing of any runners behind me. I began to wonder if they were going the right way but getting lost is pretty impossible as the path is between the river and a busy dual carriageway. As I crossed the bridge and began running down the opposite side of the river, I looked back and noticed the next runner was a few hundred yards behind me. I felt very much in the lead at the time.

After completing the first lap, I set off on the second and noticed that the runner behind me was still some distance behind. I began to think of the glory of leading from start to finish. OK, it was a multi-distance event, so that some people would be running much further than me, but that didn't matter. The last time I ran here, I got a little badge saying, 'First Finisher'. I became determined to repeat this and be the first to check-in. Lap two was good, but it started getting hotter, and my pace slowed slightly. However, I was still well in front and really enjoying it.

Lap two was completed, and I set off on number three. The third one is a little shorter for the half marathon distance to make up the final two and a half miles. As my watch ticked over the eleven miles, my legs felt incredibly heavy, and a bit of fatigue kicked in. This is the fatigue associated with my brain injury and not general tiredness from running or lack of sleep.

The voices in my head are constantly chattering away when I run, but they jumped up a gear now. Nooooooo, not now! I'm leading the pack now, and I really don't want to blow this personal victory and ruin the moment because of this damn brain of mine. I'm still in front, so just slow down and enjoy it. How long to go now? 11.25 miles done; I thought I'd done more than a quarter of a mile since last looking. Yeah, but you knew that because you've done this course before. OK, just keep going, one foot in front of the other and avoid looking at the watch. Hmm, just one quick look. Why? I have covered about ten steps since the last one.

This continued for the rest of the run. I stopped on a small bridge and walked ten steps before starting again. At the point where I was due to turn left on the shortened half marathon trail, I opened a kissing gate and looked back. There were no other runners in sight behind me. The voice now turned a little positive, and I turned back into the hotel car park, signalled a bell ringing action for the clock to be stopped and headed to the cake table with a big smile on my face. The organiser presented me with a huge Cakeathon medal and stuck the First Finisher badge on the ribbon. I grabbed a slice of cake and a drink before making my way to a rock underneath the trees and sat down to eat and recover. It was time for the imposter syndrome excuses like this was a timed event, and only a handful of us were doing the half. Also, some runners had completed shorter distances, and the marathon guy would probably finish in a much quicker time than I could do a marathon, so if he did the half, he'd beat me. Then, I had a reality check and decided to celebrate being first across the line at half distance. My CV could now read first places in a 1 mile, a 5K, a 10K and a half marathon (twice). That's a bit of personal satisfaction. These were all personal victories to me, and I'd celebrate them as much as I did when completing my first half marathon, my first marathon and the personal bests along the way even though I had reservations about mentioning first-place finishes in races as, in my eyes, running is about your own personal victories and not necessarily about winning.

As you know, I'm too modest when winning things individually so imagine my delight to be part of a first placed team recently. A team of three Conquer the Castle at Rockingham Castle in Northamptonshire. It was another timed event of six hours with 5K laps to run. This time, team competition was on the stage. Mark, from MRMAK and another club buddy, Ben, set off on our laps over the tough and challenging route. As we passed the halfway point, we realised that we were doing well and began to feel a little more competitive and started to work out how many laps we could complete in total. We did 14 laps in a time of just under 6:10, breaking the course record and finishing in first place overall. The team spirit and support for each other throughout the day was immense and was a real testament to the wonderful sport that we love.

―――

Real Life Stories From The Field - In It For The Long Run

Running has introduced me to some remarkable people, but one incredible person who springs to mind is a friend of mine at my running club called Michael. We met a few years ago when he joined, and I found him easy to talk to, as he was, like many other runners, quite humble in his achievements. He'd done lots of marathons and began talking about ultra events. It wasn't just talking though; he was actually running them. Yep, races of 50 miles and even 100+.

In 2019, while we were out on a Monday evening recovery run, I asked him what his next crazy event would be, and he casually replied, *'Oh, I've entered the JOGLE!'* After asking him for an explanation, he confirmed it was a race from John O' Groats to Lands' End, that's 860 miles from the most northern tip of Scotland to southeast England. Suddenly, I was excited but probably not as excited as Michael was.

Fast forward to 2022, after a summer club night, I caught up with my good friend and asked him to tell me his story.

'Well, the dream of doing the JOGLE started about four years ago. It was something I knew I had to do, and I finally signed up for the 2020 race. Although I trained really hard, doing long runs of 30-40 miles, there was a nagging doubt in my mind that I wouldn't finish it. I'd done numerous ultras, including 100-mile events, but this just felt different; I knew I lacked mental belief.

Three days into the race, the event was pulled due to the country going into lockdown. It was strange, but I felt a sense of relief, even though I hadn't ever told anyone about this.

The organisers kindly gave us a big discount for the following year's race so, in June 2021, I was on the start line at John O' Groats again. However, this time I had more belief and felt ready. After a week of running and walking the length of Scotland, I made it to Gretna on the border of England. Suddenly, I had a sickening feeling in my stomach, but it wasn't from anything other than the pain in my right quad muscle. I made my checkpoint and rested for the night, but it felt really sore the following morning.

Nineteen miles into day eight, I reached Penrith but had to stop. I simply couldn't carry on as the pain was too much and had to drop out of the race.

Many people have asked me how I felt, and the answer was simply devastated. I was a total wreck and in floods of tears. I called my wife, Dawn, to tell her, but I just couldn't speak. As the support car picked me up to take me back to my hotel, I immediately thought, I'm not finished with this, I'll be back next year.

Amazingly, I recovered from the injury very quickly and did the Lakeland 100-mile ultra in July, a mere six weeks later.

The following month, I suffered another ultra setback at the Ultra Trail Mont Blanc. This is an epic race with a really strict qualification. Sixty-five miles into the race, I mentally prepared myself for a massive climb as the route left Italy and entered Switzerland. Due to feeling tired and not paying full attention, I failed to notice fellow runners passing me, and I missed the strict time cut-off at the checkpoint by five minutes. Again, I was gutted.

As Christmas 2021 approached, I treated myself to a Christmas present. What more could one man wish for than an entry to the JOGLE 2022? My mind was firmly set on achieving my dream of reaching that finish line at Lands' End.

To focus on my training, I completed the Centurion Virtual event, which involved running 1,000 miles in 100 days. I ran five days a week with back-to-back runs of 15, 20 and 25 miles at the weekend. My longest solo run was 55 miles following the Northamptonshire Round, which circumnavigated the county.

I was also aware I hadn't fuelled myself properly the previous year, leaving it too long before eating in the evening. Even waiting an hour can be critical in recovery. So, I tried a new protein brand which seemed to work well in training.

Arriving at John O' Groats for the third time, I was quietly confident that in 17 days' time, I would be celebrating in Lands' End.

Day one went smoothly for me, and I was fourth out of the field of seven. Sadly, the first finisher that day had to quit for medical reasons, showing that you never know what this race will throw at you. We had our second and third dropout on day four, but you had to focus on your race and goal.

On day seven, things were going well until I felt a familiar sickly feeling in the pit of my stomach. It was like deja vu as I was running through Gretna and felt a twinge in my left knee and had to stop. This brought flashbacks of the previous year as I'd now resorted to walking and hiked ten miles from Gretna to Carlisle to the next checkpoint.

With 57 miles to cover the following day, I took painkillers and used a vibrating massage gun that I'd bought for the event in every attempt to solve the issue.

Day eight was probably the most challenging day out of the seventeen days of running, having to hike for 57 miles at just over four mph pace! That night as I was eating my evening meal, my knee kept seizing up, and I kept thinking, this is it, race over again. After taking more painkillers and sleeping like a baby, I woke up and felt no pain. I was delighted and set off with a plan to run and walk the long distance. Thankfully, my legs felt great.

After more days of running and walking, taking in the beautiful scenery and pushing from point to point, the next major mishaps occurred. On day 13, there were two of us left in the race. The route was 55 miles from Bristol to Wellington, and I set off, running the first stretch to get some early miles under my belt. My fellow runner was nowhere to be seen, so I was left alone and later found out she had to retire. That was it, there was only me left.

During that day, I made my way along a trail called the Strawberry Line. It was an old disused railway line that was straight as a die. Halfway along the flat pathway, I had a call of nature and needed to leave the path to find somewhere quiet and private to... well, you know! After some much-needed relief, I returned to the path and picked up my pace again. However, three miles later, I began to sense something wasn't quite right and realised that I'd been running in the wrong direction. After a quick call to the organiser, he confirmed this, and I now had to turn around and run another three miles back to the pitstop before getting back on track. Due to my tiredness, I ended up covering over 60 miles that day. It sounds like a really simple mistake, but I can't stress how mentally tiring this event was.

My mindset was still firmly set on achieving my goal. Despite pains in my shins, I kept going. Each day I'd get up, run for an hour, and then take walking breaks. I would be fine if my pace remained at about an average of 4mph. Each day ticked off was a day closer to the finish line.

On the last day, I knew I'd finish it. I left my hotel with a mere 30 miles to go. After a few miles, I reached Penzance and followed a series of undulating and bendy roads, needing my wits about me to avoid any cars flying around the corners.

My adrenaline rose as I realised there was only a mile to go, so I picked up my pace and began running. This is it; the finish line is in sight. I could hear some faint cheers getting louder. 'C'mon Granddad!' The emotion was rising as I could hear the voices of my grandkids, Harry, Lucy and Jessica. Their cheers were coupled with my daughter Abbi, her partner Chris, and my wonderful wife, Dawn. They ran the final steps to the Lands' End sign when I reached my JOGLE goal.

Wow, absolutely amazing! After four years of visualising this moment repeatedly in my head, it was now real. You'd think I'd be able to stop having those dreams, but it took me around four weeks to stop dreaming of running after this epic journey was complete.

The organisers presented me with a big trophy for winning the JOGLE. There was also a medal, a bunch of flowers, a massive bottle of champagne and the gift of a weekend away. That was some goodie bag for sure.

In 2019, I finished joint first in the Glendower Way ultra, over 135 miles. I crossed the line with a fellow runner I'd run with for 15 miles. The JOGLE was not only a personal victory of achievement but an event in that I finished in first place. My running time of eight days, 15 hours and 15 minutes is the fourth quickest in this race's history, and if it hadn't been for the wrong turning and extra six miles, I would be in the top three. However, I'm immensely proud. It just feels fantastic!

Having known Michael for many years, he is still humble and passionate when telling me that story, and it's one I won't tire of. It proves that we can remove obstacles from our lives and achieve what we want by simply starting with a positive mindset. What was even more jaw-dropping was the fact that not only did Michael win the race, but he did this just weeks before his 71st birthday. This story had to be shared in the Winner, Winner chapter because it's a fitting end.

I asked Michael if he ever tried to drop into conversation that he's done the JOGLE, but he replied 'no'. I knew that would be his answer, he's not the type of person to try and impress others for the sake of it. This is wonderful because many goals are personal and focusing on your own is key to achieving them.

As we left the bar where we met after our running club nights, a couple of other members were chatting about marathons. Michael asked me how many times I've done London, to which I replied four. He proudly announced that he'd done it 15 times. I put my arm around his shoulder and congratulated him for getting one over me that evening. Joking aside, he's also done more JOGLEs than me and the rest of us and is a truly inspirational person. Perhaps he should write a book (watch this space, maybe).

―――

Thoughts Running Through the Mind

'*It's not the winning; it's the taking part that counts!*' Have you heard that phrase? I bet you have many times. In fact, an elderly gentleman shouted that out to Jules when she was running the Benidorm 10K as she was enjoying the atmosphere near the back of the field.

In running, I've also heard the phrase, '*The hardest step is the first step out of the door!*' This, the most significant victory, is getting started on your mission to achieve your goal.

Think of a time when you've been your best and were really proud of your achievement. How did you celebrate your personal victories in life?

What things could you celebrate more instead of just playing them down? Perhaps it's something from the past or something that you're working towards. Great news if it's the latter. You can now use visualisation and plan how you're going to celebrate. In the chapter, *Flake Half & a Century*, I visualised my fist-pumping celebration when crossing the line at St Neots.

Sir Roger Bannister would visualise breaking the four-minute-mile barrier whilst training for this record-breaking attempt. He said that he'd wake some mornings thinking he'd actually achieved it because he'd thought about it so many times.

Visualisation is like tricking your mind into success. This was so powerful for Bannister when he broke the four-minute mile barrier on 6th May 1954.

Use your own visualisations to think about what your celebration is going to look like when you achieve your goal?

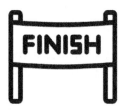

17. Congratulations on Finishing

OK, you haven't quite finished this book yet, but you're on the home straight. Can you hear the crowd cheering you along that final stretch? I sincerely thank you for reading the stories I've loved sharing with you, and I hope you'll cheer my book out loud and tell your friends about it (and perhaps leave me a nice review too).

My journey to the 100 Half Marathon Club was long. It began in 2007 and ended in 2021, spanning 14 years. In truth, it's possible to achieve this much quicker, of course. I've met people at events who have done 52 in 52 weeks and even more. However, thanks to the length of time it's taken me, it's allowed me to see such a significant change in the sport of running.

I remember seeing the first London Marathon on television as a young child in 1981. Back then, entrants had to post off their entry form and wait and see if their cheque had been cashed to know if they were in. The race itself was a monumental feat of human endurance that so few people could ever consider achieving themselves.

Around 20,000 people were reported to have entered, and just over 7,000 started the race, with some 800 dropping out on the course. Nowadays, it's believed that up to half a million people enter the event, and well over 55,000 are invited to the start line. That, in itself, shows a massive change in the popularity and inclusivity of running.

Since my journey in the sport began, and I moved on from that cotton running vest and black running trainers, running has exploded. Let me share a few final thoughts on what works for me in running, plus some quirky observations about the sport. There are also a few tips for newer runners looking to get started or progress.

What to Choose

There are more and more events to choose from nowadays. It could be possible to race on a Saturday morning, find another event in the afternoon and do another on Sunday if you're mad enough. More events are beginner-friendly and welcoming to all ages and abilities.

When Paul Sinton-Hewitt lined up with a few fellow runners to compete in a five-kilometre time trial in 2004, I bet he never imagined that there would now be over 2,000 parkrun events worldwide. In my opinion, it must be one of the biggest and best volunteer-led sporting events on the planet and gives the public many choices. I probably have a couple of dozen parkruns within 25 miles of my home.

In addition to parkrun, many running clubs and companies put on events of all distances worldwide. When I began running, there were only a small number of races locally. Northampton didn't have a half marathon or a marathon, so it meant travelling a little further.

So how do new runners choose their first event? Like most things, there isn't a one size fits all answer. Mine was a big, mass participation event, namely the Great North Run. I was drawn in by the big crowds and the atmosphere. On the other hand, Jules likes to run abroad where she doesn't know anyone because she's a little more self-conscious. Of course, parkrun is an ideal and safe place to start too. Families can join in many fun runs and run or walk together.

Full Kit

I may have evolved from those aforementioned black trainers and cotton vest and bought some decent running shoes. However, the sport can still be simple and affordable to kit yourself out. If you ask any runner their advice, one of the first things they'll say is to buy a decent pair of shoes, so that's probably the biggest outlay. I've mentioned that I'm not one for the latest brands and significant expenses and always find a good deal online. I guess I have the advantage of knowing what shoes and the support I need, but it's a good idea to go to a specialist running shop and speak to an expert to ensure you get the right shoes. Having a gait analysis is key here. Most top running shops will check out how your feet land as you run and advise on the support and structure of the footwear. Make sure this act is carried out by an expert and not a sales rep. It's simple but be aware that marketing is also clever by influencing you into spending more money.

Aside from shoes, we runners love our race t-shirts. They're like a badge of honour when you proudly wear them to show off the event we've just completed, just like I wear my 100 Half Marathon t-shirt. Of course, many events give medals, but I've not yet experienced any running buddies running with those around their neck in a training run. The t-shirt is more practical.

Many events give out technical t-shirts, which are great for absorbing sweat. The running family is also comfortable with sweating and not looking your most glamorous after a run.

I've done a few events where the goodie bag has included some tremendous running socks. Again, I'm a big fan of getting a few decent pairs for my feet to be comfortable. Add a decent pair of shorts, and we're ready to go. My favourite pair are bright yellow. Running can be colourful.

The Price to Pay

Running can be inexpensive, but it can also cost a lot of money if you allow it to. Of course, the kit can be reasonable or highly priced, and so can events.

When I began running, the first local races I entered cost much less than £10 but entry fees have increased over the years. More events and companies are organising races now, with this comes higher costs with chip timing, for example. In my early events, my time was sometimes written down by a volunteer holding a clipboard. The convenience of chip activation is worth the price for both runners and organisers.

Lots of events mean competition, and competition to get people to enter equals advertising costs. These then have to be factored into the entry fees. We then enter the race online, so there are website costs and transaction fees for paying by card. We mustn't forget all the health and safety processes, liability insurance and road closure costs.

I'm always on the hunt for a bargain and look closely at race entry fees. If it's too expensive, then I generally don't enter. However, I don't mind paying a little more for events run by small independent companies that host the events themselves and put a lot of time and effort into making them happen.

It's also possible to do free events too. As mentioned, many times in this book, you don't get freer and more well organised than the weekly parkrun events. Also, by looking around, there are some great low-cost races. I have paid between £5 and over £50 to enter events. Some events are more, especially if the host's costs are higher. Recently, I saw a race that offered an interest free option to pay for the entry. Running a seven-day ultra across the Sahara Dessert could be thousands of pounds, so you must commit to a good training plan should you be brave enough to enter.

Scenery and Surroundings

I've mentioned many times that one thing I love about running is the scenery and locations it can take you to. If you drive from A to B, you generally spend more time looking at the road ahead. Well, at least I sincerely hope you do. That means you miss a lot of the journey. By running, you get to see more and quicker than you would walking (I love both, of course).

My favourite races have taken me around stately homes like Blenheim Palace in Oxfordshire and Ashridge Estate in Berkshire. I've run along the coastlines of England as well as those races abroad. I did two more races in

Lanzarote a few weeks before writing this chapter. One was a Disco Night Run, a colourful and musical 10K around the island's capital. It took in a lovely old harbour, and a firework display was on the first lap. That was special! The other event was my first attempt at an obstacle race near the island's airport. Probably something I wouldn't have normally tried back home. Running up a mountain in the Highland Games was a highlight too. Beach running, forest running, rural routes, big cities and even around castles, as long as you're safe, there's a route for everyone.

Techno, Techno

Do you have a mate who has to have the latest gadget? Perhaps that's you? Also, if you're like me and love stats, you'll love running. Now, I can bore Jules silly with my race splits by telling her which mile was my fastest and which one had the killer hill, and I can prove that with an elevation graph downloaded to an app from my GPS running watch. Put me in a room full of fellow runners after an event, and I have a captive audience as we all swap our stats for hours.

Gadgets sound expensive, but you have Mr Bargain on your side here. I've owned a range of running watches over the years, but the main thing that's important to me is recording my pace, distance and time while running. This can be achieved with an inexpensive watch. The beauty of my latest watch is it was a hand-me-down from a running buddy who'd upgraded. I still thank my mate Bob for his kindness and generosity.

Great news for newer runners or those on a budget, this can be recorded free with apps on a mobile phone, and there are many to choose from. Looking at a phone while running is a little more challenging though.

A final observation on that point. Running does carry a warning that runners will become obsessed with rounding their training runs up to the nearest mile. Newer runners give puzzled looks as fully grown adults slowly plod around in a circle or up and down a path attempting to get their distance from 5.89 miles to record exactly six miles. Running friends, hold your hands up and admit that you do this.

More About Lines and Less About Times

In my time running, I've seen many new runners do their first few events and then get caught by the PB bug. As their early fitness builds, their times drop, and they record PB after PB. What happens when the PBs dry up? Unfortunately, some runners start to lose interest and fall away, and Sharky's earlier story was an excellent example of this.

I've heard the phrase, '*More about lines and less about times*' a lot in running, and it sums up the wonder of the sport. Getting to the finish line is a gift and something to be cherished. I'm always on the lookout for new and exciting challenges. These could be random, quirky events like the Los Pocillos Obstacle Race in Lanza, mentioned above. There are different distances to try and even challenges you could create yourself. I've done parkruns where I've started at the very back to see how much time I can make up or how many places I can gain. This is also very sociable because I sometimes run with a friend I find on the course.

Another beauty of running is, as you pass a birthday, your previous times can be wiped clean, and you can start chasing new age PBs. Most, but not all people, generally slow down as they get older, so new age category personal bests can be a huge motivator.

Like-minded Crazy Friends

OK, we're not crazy, but a lot of my non-running friends use that word to describe my running pursuits. A running friend sent me a message that read, *'Happy birthday to a crazy but lovely guy.'* What a nice description!

Why not hang out with some like-minded friends? The local running community here is wonderful, but the great thing is, wherever I run in the world, it's exactly the same. Everyone seems so friendly and encouraging.

I've mentioned my running club, Northampton Road Runners, many times throughout this book. Our ethos is to offer members a safe and comfortable environment and, most of all, enjoy themselves. It's a really friendly club where we aim to help people achieve their goals. It's also introduced me to friends with whom I've formed lifelong bonds through running.

There are many groups that newer runners can join, from beginners' groups to progression groups. I've seen more and more varieties of groups pop up in recent years. These range from female running groups to Couch to 5K and mental health talk groups. There are also groups for serious athletes too. At our club, we have pop-up groups that will focus on training for a particular event or introduce members to something new like trail running their fist marathon, for example.

I always feel that the best way to become better at something is to find a group of people who are striving for similar goals and share the journey. However, if someone is a little more self-conscious, running is something you can enjoy in the quiet and tranquillity of your own company too.

Oh, and don't forget the cake.

Yeah, now I may have mentioned cake several times throughout this book. Can I just clarify that not every event will give you cake. I don't want you to enter an event with high expectations and come and hunt me down when you get a strange goodie bag gift like a bag of salt, for example. However, lots of my running friends enjoy the fitness benefits enough to enjoy a treat now and again. Go on, treat yourself (in moderation, of course).

Then there are t-shirts and goodie bags. My cupboard has far too many race memento shirts, but I try to wear them all for running or everyday life. You can usually tell a runner - they typically wear a race event t-shirt and an old pair of running shoes in public.

Bling, Bling

Olympic athletes get gold medals for winning the Olympic Games, and the great news here is, lots of events give medals too. Even better, you don't have to win to get one. Amazing!

Like t-shirts, I have a box full of medals, probably worth a small fortune in scrap metal if I wanted to cash in.

———

Stories From the Field - Runners Advice

For the final *Stories from the Field*, I asked fellow runners what advice they'd give to their former selves if they were to begin running again. Amazingly, the tips they shared are helpful for all runners of all abilities, whether they're beginners or experienced. There are so many, and here is a shortlist below:

- At events, smile for the cameras and always thank the volunteers.
- Don't always worry too much about times. Whether it's your first race, first half or marathon, or you've been running for years make sure you enjoy your running. If you are going for a time and you don't get it, avoid beating yourself up. There's always another event.
- Try to relax in the build-up to events. It's easy to get nervous, but if you've put the training miles in, you'll be in good shape (and if you haven't, get around the course and enjoy it).
- If you're training for a marathon, don't skimp on the long runs or walks. Time on your feet is critical. It doesn't matter how slowly you're running, just get used to being on your feet for long periods.
- Find some running buddies to get you through tough days when it may be bad weather or you don't feel like going out of the door. The first step is usually the hardest, and you rarely regret going for a run.
- Follow a training plan but make sure you enjoy it. Don't feel guilty if you miss a day. Please make sure you have fun without overthinking it. Don't stress too much about missing runs, just try your best to hit the weekly goals. Also, slowly increase each week instead of making big jumps in distance. This will only lead to injury.

- Make sure you fuel yourself properly for a race. This is key in both the build-up and on the day itself. Also, experiment with what works well for you. There's nothing worse than trying something new on race day and finding it doesn't work. Also, train in the kit you plan to wear on the day, don't save new trainers, underwear, socks etc., for the big event, make sure they are comfortable beforehand. Also, use anti-chafe on anything that might rub together and always double-knot your shoelaces.
- Try to avoid putting too much pressure on yourself to achieve a time, especially if it's your first event. You never know how the day will go with nerves and excitement. Enjoy the day and be in the moment.
- It's important not to overdo things, as injuries and other setbacks can always get in the way. I've learned the hard way in the past that pushing yourself too hard for too long to attain those PBs can end in injury and leave you on the sidelines for weeks, months or even years. Also, be mindful of the age factor, as unfortunately, none of us are getting any younger. My mentality in recent years is to slow down, take it easy and really, really enjoy my running. That way, I've ended up running more mileage than ever before with fewer injuries.
- Don't worry if you need to take a walking break or stop for a drink. There's no shame and it will most likely benefit you in the long run.
- Incorporate cross-training into your plan. Perhaps going to the gym and doing a core and leg strength included. Pilates or yoga is fantastic too. Also, make sure you rest too. Rest days are equally important.
- Find an event with a nice goody bag, t-shirt, medal and a good atmosphere. If you're not into material gifts, find one that you'll enjoy.
- If you're a beginner and things start to ache, don't worry; you're using muscles you probably haven't used before.

Behind the Scenes - The Race Director's View
Now I wouldn't have been able to complete my 100 Half Marathon journey without the dedication of hundreds of people working tirelessly behind the scenes to put these events on.

Being on the committee of a running club who have arranged races in the past, it gave me an insight to how big a job this can be. So, how about we finish with someone who not only has a passion for the sport as an athlete but also as an event organiser. Naturally, I became good friends with Simon Hollis, Race Director of Go Beyond Challenge, who set up the Northampton Half Marathon. Simon is an Ultra Marathon Runner and was kind enough to share his story.

'Military life as a young man rarely leaves you without some damage, either physically mentally or both, it's the chance we take. These things often catch up you up when you least expect them. A diagnosis is often a blessing to help you understand what is happening to you and why you feel like you do.

I guess the job as a race director is least suited to my PTSD diagnosis with lots of stress around race day and the constant challenge of obstacles in the way, however, resilience is a word much talked about these days and having been in some dark places I have certainly learnt the value of this. I really have empathy with the worried runners on the start line! I have endured some of the toughest footraces on Earth mainly through my suborn nature and my deep-seated desire never to give up. We all fall into the same trap when going to events, races, gigs etc. where we forget the work that goes into making your day the best it can be and even sorting problems out that you never knew existed. Despite organising a whole bunch of well-established events, it always surprises me the amount of work involved in keeping everything up to date and striving to make things better. Never forget to smile and say thank you to the events team!

So, what made me get into arranging race events? One October night a few years ago an accountant friend called me and said that they had a client who was selling his event management business and she thought of me. I decided it was now or never so took the plunge.

The hardest thing about setting up events can be the greed of venues and their lack of support for events. Some councils, trusts and private businesses all see a busy event and assume that the organisers are making loads of money and that they should have some of that.

Runners can sometimes underestimate what goes into arranging event toos. I think it's the infrastructure we build around events: medical support, route planning, vehicles, set up teams, break down teams, sweeper teams and the level of communication that goes on. But the most important thing is that they don't see all of this and they just have a great day. However, most of them respect the work of the marshal team and rightly so.

Running always throws up unexpected amusing moments and a couple of examples spring to mind.

At the Thames Trot a few years ago, I was approached before the race by a girl who was an Instagram influencer and wanted to take part in the event in exchange for sharing her experience with her many thousands of followers. She was petite and very nicely presented for a 48-mile ultra-marathon and I did think I would see her getting out of the sweeper bus at the finish. Anyway, lots of gnarly guys crossed the line covered in mud and complaining and crying about how hard it was, then in the distance appeared my influencer skipping towards the finish with a big smile on her face only to announce that she had a lovely day end really enjoyed the experience!

The Country to Capital had to be re-routed one year as they dug up the road we planned to run along. We had to use a footpath just before the roadworks where you had to duck under a tree branch that had grown across which was also the location of the checkpoint. During the race Deano, the marshal at the checkpoint, called me to say that a man had appeared with a chain saw and he wanted to cut the tree down in the middle of the race. It transpired that Deano calculated the gap between the lead group and the following pack and told the guy that's how long he had. Suffice to say it was the quickest tree he ever cut down and the runners were unaware of the drama that had unfolded.'

What a fabulous insight into the life of a major event organiser. Personally, I've always been polite enough to thank people, especially volunteers at events. This has made me even more determined to find the organisers and personally thank them for their hard work.

Thoughts Running Through the Mind

Here we are, we've now crossed the line and we've come to the end of the book. It's time for a few final thoughts.

You've seen many analogies linking running and life together in the stories throughout this book, and it's true that when you reach the finish line of a goal, life doesn't stop.

My life is on a much more even keel now, but I'm still on my journey. The old cliche says it's not a sprint, it's a marathon. That's very true to life! Yes, I still suffer from anxiety and panic attacks, but they are fewer now. Thanks to the support and coping mechanisms shared by some wonderful people, I've managed to come to terms with the new me, new being used loosely as it's been ten years since my accident. Like running, I'm always looking for fresh strategies and goals to achieve in life. Being in personal development, always striving to learn new things and seek exciting challenges is key to becoming fulfilled.

It's time for a post-run debrief! So, go back to the thoughts sections in the book and take an in-depth look at your goals and the things you perhaps wrote down (or made a mental note of) and revisit them.

I practiced and taught goal setting for many years and could write a whole book on the topic. However, let's summarise a simple process to follow.

First, set the goal, without a target, you have nothing to aim for. Next, make plans to move forward to achieve the goal. If the goal is big, break those steps down into smaller bite-sized chunks. Remember to make small, consistent steps. It's the small actions that add up to the big results.

Also, ask yourself what tools you'll need and who can help you. If the tools are expensive, you may have a sub-goal to make a savings plan, and this becomes another step to break into bite-sized chunks. A tool could be knowledge. I won't hide the fact that I've read many personal development and running books in the lead up to writing Half Man, Half Marathon.

The who is simple. Who's an expert in the field of the goal that you're setting? If they've achieved it, ask them how. If they're not easily accessible then study them, read their biography on how they achieved their success.

Another key step is to set a date. Having a date in mind makes the goal real and solid. It will help you to visualise its achievement. Remember, dates can be changed should things not go to plan.

One final point is to note your why. The why can arguably be one of the most powerful keys to your success. Let's face it, if you don't know why you're wanting to achieve something then it's going to be difficult to remain focused on the end goal.

It's time to collect your virtual medal and keep running towards those life goals. Good luck, and I wish you every success. Keep on running.

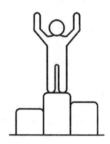

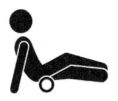

Cool Down and Recovery Time

After the event, it's really important to take time to rest and recover. This is an ideal moment to reflect on and enjoy your accomplishments. Now you've enjoyed my story, let's take a look at your journey. Whether you're running your first Couch to 5K, first parkrun, inaugural 10k, half marathon or even marathon, celebrate all of your achievements along the way.

If you're looking to get started on your journey to the 100 Half Marathon or 100 Marathon Club, my advice is to keep track of your races as you go along. Also, make a note of the web link from the event's resulwts page as this will save you a lot of time in the future. You can also submit your results as you go along. The 100 Half Marathon Club has milestones at 25, 50, and 100.

Take a look at the website www.100halfmarathonclub.co.uk and this will give you all the information you need to know. The organisers are super helpful and will answer any questions if you drop them a line.

If you're a self-confessed statto like me, then you may enjoy my list of hundred half marathons that took me to that magic milestone. Enjoy them on the following page and don't forget to check out some of the brilliant events listed.

A Journey of Race Stats

1	The Great North Run	30/09/07	1:59:37
2	London Half Marathon at Silverstone	09/03/08	1:49:59
3	Bournemouth Bay Run	30/03/08	1:47:00
4	Cransley Hospice Half	21/09/08	1:45:36
5	The Great North Run	04/10/08	1:48:21
6	Bedford Harriers Half Marathon	14/12/08	1:43:31
7	Milton Keynes Half Marathon	08/03/09	1:40:50
8	London Half Marathon at Silverstone	15/03/09	1:39:42
*	Ashby 20	22/03/09	3:13:57
9	Cransley Hospice Half	20/09/09	1:44:41
10	Royal Parks Half Marathon	11/10/09	1:39:45
11	Milton Keynes Half Marathon	07/03/10	1:38:02
12	London Half Marathon at Silverstone	14/03/10	1:42:40
13	Water Of Life Half Marathon	21/03/10	1:41:03
14	Bournemouth Bay Run	28/03/10	1:43:40
15	Dunstable Downs Half Marathon Challenge	12/09/10	1:53:15
16	Cransley Hospice Half	19/09/10	1:41:08
17	Charwood Hills Race	06/02/11	2:06:32
18	London Half Marathon at Silverstone	06/03/11	1:35:28
*	Ashby 20	13/03/11	3:11:47
*	Oakley 20	27/03/11	3:10:44
19	Bournemouth Bay Run	03/04/11	1:37:34
20	Alexander The Great Half Marathon	12/06/11	1:39:07
21	Colworth Marathon Challenge	26/06/11	1:51:15
22	Adderbury Shires & Spires	09/07/11	1:44:11
23	Dunstable Downs Half Marathon Challenge	11/09/11	1:45:25
24	Belvoir Challenge	25/02/12	2:19:48
25	Berkhamsted Half	04/03/12	1:40:45
**	The Grizzly	11/03/12	4:13:53
26	Bournemouth Bay Run	01/04/12	1:34:06
27	Otmoor Challenge	09/06/12	1:46:58
28	Adderbury Shires & Spires	14/07/12	1:48:11
29	Charwood Hills Race	03/02/13	2:19:43
30	Belvoir Challenge	23/02/13	2:18:19
31	Berkhamsted Half	03/03/13	1:33:17
*	The Grizzly	10/03/13	4:03:53
*	Ashby 20	17/03/13	2:45:48
32	Otmoor Challenge	01/06/13	1:36:56
33	Desborough Half	30/06/13	1:43:39
34	Adderbury Shires & Spires	13/07/13	1:51:03
35	The Beast	01/09/13	1:51:18
36	Northampton Half Marathon	22/09/13	2:02:16
37	Blenheim Half Marathon	06/10/13	1:35:58
38	Lode Half	03/11/13	1:36:47
39	The Dirt Half	16/11/13	1:39:28
40	Bedford Harriers Half Marathon	08/12/13	1:37:15
41	Berkhamsted Half	02/03/14	1:37:13
*	The Grizzly	09/03/14	4:38:35

42	Northampton Running Festival	20/04/14	1:43:32
43	Shakespeare Half	27/04/14	1:38:33
44	Milton Keynes Festival of Running	05/05/14	1:36:59
45	Otmoor Challenge	07/06/14	1:58:53
46	Adderbury Shires & Spires	12/07/14	1:50:15
47	Northampton Half Marathon	14/09/14	1:36:41
48	Bedford Harriers Half Marathon	08/12/14	1:35:44
49	Berkhamsted Half	01/03/15	1:38:53
50	Battlefield Half	08/03/15	1:35:08
51	Obelisk Obble	14/03/15	1:59:05
52	Northampton Running Festival	05/04/15	1:43:40
53	Bournemouth Bay Run	12/04/15	1:34:39
54	Milton Keynes Festival of Running	04/05/15	1:32:33
55	Farthingstone Foot Fest	06/06/15	2:33:00
56	Rugby Half	13/07/15	1:37:06
57	Kimbolton Half	16/08/15	1:35:22
58	Northampton Half Marathon	06/09/15	1:31:47
59	The Great North Run	13/09/15	1:34:11
60	Bournemouth Bay Run Marathon Fest	04/10/15	1:31:54
61	Lode Half	01/11/15	1:30:12
62	St Neots Riverside Half Marathon	15/11/15	1:34:06
63	Lanzarote Half	12/12/15	1:39:39
64	Harborough Running Festival	11/06/16	1:36:50
65	Adderbury Shires & Spires	10/07/16	1:47:12
66	Northampton Half Marathon	04/09/16	1:33:31
67	Feurteventura International Dunas Half	30/10/16	1:56:32
68	Charwood Hills Race	05/02/17	2:42:21
69	Welly Trail Half Marathon	19/02/17	2:22:34
70	Stanwick Lakes Half	12/03/17	1:36:18
71	Belvoir Half	07/04/17	1:49:10
72	Stanwick Lakes Half	11/06/17	1:36:10
73	Colworth Marathon Challenge	25/06/17	1:40:54
74	Kimbolton Half	20/08/17	1:39:47
75	Northampton Half Marathon	03/09/17	1:35:25
76	Blenheim Half Marathon	01/10/17	1:38:45
77	Goa River Half Marathon	10/12/17	2:04:18
78	Welly Trail Half Marathon	18/02/18	2:07:17
79	Belvoir Challenge	24/02/18	2:21:46
*	Milton Keynes 20	11/03/18	3:01:03
80	Obelisk Obble	25/03/18	2:21:00
81	Otmoor Challenge	02/06/18	1:51:40
82	Palma Media Maraton	14/10/18	1:44:20
83	Dunstable Downs Half Marathon Challenge	01/09/19	1:45:30
84	Northampton Half Marathon	29/09/19	1:41:45
85	Benidorm Half	29/02/20	1:42:51
86	Clipston Trail Half	27/09/20	1:53:08
87	Water Of Life Half Marathon	18/10/20	1:46:26
88	Leicestershire Half Marathon	18/04/21	1:38:36
89	Saxon Shore Olympic Challenge	01/05/21	1:45:50
90	St Albans Half Marathon	13/06/21	1:49:47
91	Enigma Running Shaken Not Stirred	03/07/21	1:47:39

92	Big Bear Salcey Summer Challenge	08/07/21	2:05:44
93	Cransley Hospice Half	19/09/21	1:42:11
94	Northampton Half Marathon	26/09/21	1:43:18
95	Run Silverstone Half Marathon	10/10/21	1:54:33
96	Big Bear Rainbow Challenge	13/10/21	2:02:31
97	Water Of Life Half Marathon	24/10/21	1:48:07
98	Baldock Beast	31/10/21	1:54:15
99	Zig Zag Remberance Run	14/11/21	1:46:42
100	St Neots Riverside Half Marathon	21/11/21	1:38:22
109	Zig Zag Christmas Canter	05/12/21	2:03:09
110	Benidorm Half	05/03/22	1:41:10
111	Draycote Water Half Marathon	13/03/22	1:58:41
112	Loughborough Half Marathon	03/04/22	1:45:46
113	Saxon Shore Northampton Cakeathon	16/04/22	1:51:23
114	Northants Shires and Spires (tail runner)	15/05/22	3:36:02
115	Conquer the Castle	23/07/22	2:10:57

* I didn't count 20 mile events until I'd completed 100 half marathons

Useful websites:

UK 100 Half Marathon Club - 100halfmarathonclub.co.uk

UK 100 Marathon Club - 100marathonclub.org.uk

parkrun UK - parkrun.org.uk

Go Beyond Sport (including the Northampton Half Marathon) - gobeyondchallenge.com

Phoenix Running - phoenixrunning.co.uk

Running Tales Podcast - stepforwardwithlewis.com/runningtales

Northampton Road Runners - northamptonroadrunners.co.uk

Cassandra Farren – cassandrafarren.com (book mentoring)

Kennedy Authors – kennedyauthors.co.uk

Future Toolbox (our personal development business) - futuretoolbox.co.uk

Other Titles and Resources

What The Hell Just Happened?

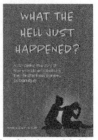

Have you experienced a challenge in your life that has pushed you to your limit? From brain injury to breast cancer and bereavement What the Hell Just Happened is the compelling, true story of how a couple stayed strong in the face of adversity. At times, they were beaten, battered and broken, their mental health and resilience was tested to the max. Find out how the phrase, 'holiday of a lifetime' took a whole new meaning for Mark and Jules Kennedy. Their story will not only make you laugh and cry, it will inspire you to never give up, no matter what life throws at you.

Anxiety, depression and mental health issues are important subjects at the forefront of people's minds. This book will help you to understand that at times, it's ok not to be ok.

Don't Get Your Neck Tattooed

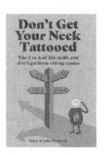

Growing up is tough! Worried about what your future self will be? Unsure of how to become the person who you really want to become? Faced with choices, pressure and responsibilities that don't seem to make a lot of sense? Ever find yourself lacking motivation? Feel that life has little direction? Do you dream about a great life but have no idea how to make it real? If your answer is yes to any of this, then you are not alone. Well, today you can make a change and begin your journey to make it happen.

Meet Milo, a regular teen who goes on a journey through the "Z to A of Life", where each letter stands for essential life habits that will help bring you success, stressing that 'this is how life can be if you want it to be'. He doesn't go backwards but sometimes life doesn't go in the order we expect it to. By creating positive mindsets, developing great habits and learning from successful people, you can now turn dreams into realities.

Whether you're a teenager with ambition, a parent or teacher looking to help turn a teen from downbeat to upbeat or an adult who wants to get life back on track, "Don't Get Your Neck Tattooed" is here to help.

We All Follow The Cobblers......Over Land & Sea

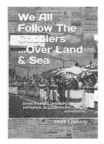

I'm a Northampton Town fan but whoever you follow, you will be able to resonate with these stories of humour, loyalty, desperation, joy and despair.

Read about the fan who messed up his chance to play for the club. Hear what happened to a fan's item of clothing whilst celebrating a goal. Meet the fans who never miss a game no matter what. Re-live a 7-0 defeat at Scunthorpe or a 5-0 loss at Burnley on a cold Tuesday night. Find out what the opposition fans think when you're playing them.

The beauty of football is that every fan has a story to tell. A story of glory, a story of pain. A story of frustration or a story of fun. Come and join me on a trip down memory lane of life supporting a lower league club.

Originally written in 2008, this is a republished version of the original memories.

Smarten Your Study

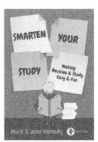

Smarten Your Study shows ways how to make revision and study, easy and fun! Do you find studying hard? Is it sometimes boring? Is it hard because it's boring or even boring because it's hard? Many students find it difficult to stay focused and get stressed out to the max by their workloads?

By opening the Future Toolbox and finding our study tools, we can help. This interactive book provides simple and fun ideas to enhance independent learning, study and revision. The aim is to help students to get into the right mindset to prepare for SATS/mocks/exams or complete vital coursework. We share tools and techniques which help to make the boring stuff fun, the hard stuff easier and turn the 'I can't' into 'I can'! With proven memory techniques, Smarten Your Study will help to create positive study habits. By having a little more fun, you will ultimately build up resilience, relieve stress and lead on a path to success.

Titles are available at **www.kennedyauthors.co.uk** plus Amazon and Kindle Unlimited.

Acknowledgements

So here we are at the end of the book you know that the bit where you say thank you to everybody who has done so much for you.

I'm going to start with the most important person in my life, that's my wife Jules, who's been there for me every step of the way, literally. Without her supporting me with my crazy running challenges and cheering me on many events, I probably would have even had the belief to get started. Of course, she's always been there to pick me up when I've been feeling very low.

Then there's the running community, starting with all my friends being Northampton Road Runners who are the most supportive people in the running world. In fact, it's the greatest running club in the world! And that's no exaggeration!

Craig Lewis who not only read the advanced manuscript but also proofread the whole thing for me out of the goodness of his heart. Craig, I'm indebted to you for your kindness. And here's a quick plug for his and his wife's podcast running tales and their brilliant personal training company Step Forward With Lewis.

Simon Hollis, of Go Beyond Sports for, not only given me the amazing Northampton Half Marathon and many other local events but for his passion and dedication to the running community and also reading and endorsing this book.

Rik Vercoe of Pheonix Running for the 100 Half Marathon Club which gave me the goal and for the kind words of endorsement.

To all the runners who shared their stories in this book and inspired you all, myself included. Thank you, Jodie TF, Sharky, Paula Solomon, Daniel Nikel, Darren Swales, John Gibbins, David Caldwell, Ben Malia, Michael Williams and, of course, Mark Rose, the other half of the MRMAK partnership.

To those who shared the short anecdotes with me in person or on social media. Now, I've tried to get you all in here so, here goes: Laura, Jason, Lesley, Theresa, Dan, Mark, Andy, Pete, Bob, Steve, Roger, Rebecca, Natasha, Jane, Simon, John, Rob, Richard, Chloe, Sue, Bex, Michelle, Becci, Joanne, Nicola, Kathy, Chrissy, James, Darren, Christopher, Chris, Guy and Vicki (phew). You're all amazing!

To Sally Wood for helping Jules and I with proofreading and opinions on the book (plus for being such a good friend). Also, to Owen Jones for advanced reading too.

Yet again to Cassandra Farren for helping with the construction of the story and mentoring me throughout writing the manuscript.

The team at Admin and More for helping with the production and marketing of the book. So, Elizabeth Wright (for running an amazing company), Elise Jenkins (for designing a brilliant cover and typesetting the manuscript, Sharon Bornheim (for being a master proof-reader and editor) and Emma O'Dea (for helping with marketing and creation). You're all amazing, wonderful people and we're so lucky to have you on board.

I have to shout out to all the race organisers and volunteers for giving us events to run. I've included a list of my races so, look them up and enter one of their events.

Finally, to anyone who's listened politely when I've been talking about running and stats.

Testimonials

'Half-man, Half-Marathon' is a fascinating look into the life of a runner - why they do the seemingly crazy challenges and distances they do, and what makes running so special.

Told through the experiences of author Mark Kennedy, who has battled against a life-changing brain injury to complete 100 half marathons, the book is a fascinating mix of running stories and a self-help manual.

Mark combines his own story with those of a cast of other runners, who have achieved everything from overcoming major life events to completing incredible challenges such as running 100 marathons or winning the 860-mile John O'Groats to Lands' End race.

If you love running, you're going to love this book.'

Craig Lewis: Producer and presenter of the Running Tales Podcast

"What kind of man takes on the challenge of 100 half marathons? What kind of man suffers personal and family challenges and still does 100 half marathons? Mark's book is both inspirational and funny and shows us all how willpower, hope and the sense of being part of something special can overcome all"

Simon Hollis: Race Director at Go Beyond Challenge and Ultra Marathon Runner

Mark writes a very open and honest account of his personal journey to 100 Half Marathons and beyond. This book tells the story of Mark's own battle following a brain injury, not just with running, but with life in general and the struggle he's faced with his own mental well-being. The ups and downs of real life are interwoven with the highs and lows of running with some wonderfully uplifting stories of the running events that Mark completed on his way to the magic 100.

Half Man, Half Marathon covers topics that will resonate with both new and experienced runners alike and also draws in real-life stories from other runners out in the field, as well as sharing plenty of useful hints and tips in every chapter. This book is very much about the journey and the people Mark met along the way, and what a journey it is.

Rik Vercoe: Ultramarathon Runner and Guinness World Record Holder (10 Marathons 10 Days), Chairman and Founder of the 100 Half Marathon Club

---